Fortschritte der Onkologie · Band 4

DNA Repair and Cancer Research

Fortschritte der Onkologie · Band 4

DNA Repair and Cancer Research

Edited by

A. Graffi, Member of Academy of Sciences,
Professor Dr. med., emerit. Director, Institute of Cancer Research,
Academy of Sciences, GDR

E. Magdon, Dr. rer. nat. habil.,
Head of Department, Institute of Cancer Research,
Academy of Sciences, GDR

Th. Matthes, Professor Dr. med.,
emerit. Director, Robert Rössle Clinic, Institute of Cancer Research,
Academy of Sciences, GDR

St. Tanneberger, Professor Dr. med. habil. Dr. rer. nat.,
Director, Institute of Cancer Research,
Academy of Sciences, GDR

AKADEMIE-VERLAG · BERLIN
1979

Erschienen im Akademie-Verlag, DDR-108 Berlin, Leipziger Straße 3—4

Lizenznummer: 202 · 100/513/79
Einband und Schutzumschlag: Rolf Kunze
Gesamtherstellung: VEB Druckhaus „Maxim Gorki", 74 Altenburg
Bestellnummer: 762 396 9 (2165/4) · LSV 2705
Printed in the GDR
DDR 48,— M

Contents

Introduction

E. MAGDON

Institute of Cancer Research, Academy of Sciences of German Democratic Republic, Berlin-Buch

The history of DNA repair in the past 15 years since the first reports of SETLOW and CARRIER (1964), BOYCE and HOWARD-FLANDERS (1964), PETTIJOHN and HANAWALT (1964) induced a lot of optimistic hopes to find a key for several unsolved problems in biology and medicine. These first studies of DNA repair processes in bacteria opened up new fields in microbiological genetics, evolution and mutagenesis but the importance of these results for medical sciences could not be assessed because it was not clear whether or not mammalian cells had similar repair systems since DNA repair was not found at first in Chinese hamster cells (SETLOW 1966).

First evidence for repair processes in mammalian cells was given by RASMUSSEN and PAINTER (1964), who reported that after irradiation with ultraviolet light all the nuclei in a culture of human HeLa cells were in DNA synthesis, which was in contrast to the 25—30% found in unirradiated cells.

Progress in the method of alkaline sucrose gradient analysis first introduced for bacteria by McGRATH and WILLIAMS (1966) and quickly adapted for analysis of mammalian cells by LETT et al. (1967) and especially the observation of CLEAVER (1968) that cells from patients with the rare genetic skin disorder, Xeroderma pigmentosum (X.p.), were defective in the excision repair pathway by which UV damage to DNA is repaired, inaugurated new prospects in oncology because the high level of actinic skin cancer is the outstanding clinical symptom of this disease.

Further studies showed that the main biochemical defect in X.p. cells occurs at an initial step of excision repair (CLEAVER 1969; SETLOW et al. 1969; BOOTSMA et al. 1970) and induced the conclusion that carcinogenesis in X.p. patients may be the result of somatic mutation caused by unrepaired DNA damage and the wider possibility exists that other forms of carcinogenesis may depend upon the same or similar principles. So the idea was put forward that excision repair is one of the cell's defences against mutation and carcinogenesis, following the interpretation that the high skin tumour incidence of X.p. patients indicates that it is the excision process which removes pyrimidine dimers as the carcinogenic stimulus.

At the Inaugural Meeting of the newly formed Section of Oncology of the Royal Society of Medicine London, HADDOW (1971) advanced the hypothesis that defects or delays in repair "may underlie the slow growth of fibroids and other benign tumours, and that greater and successive degrees of deficiency in repair may account in step-wise fashion for slowly-growing malignant tumours and for rapidly-growing malignant tumours stage by stage to the limits of anaplasia. In some such way it is likely that we now find ourselves approaching a new and unified comprehension of the wide gamut of proliferative and hypertrophic conditions ranging from the physiological at one extreme to the most highly pathological at the other".

This hypothesis to explain the process of malignant growth was not accepted in view of the observations that normal repair occurs in many malignant cells and in some X.p. patients (CLEAVER 1970 a, b; BURK et al. 1971 a, b; CLEAVER 1972; MAGDON and GUMMEL 1972).

In the meantime more than 60 patients with X.p. have been reported, DNA repair has been analysed and evidence for genetic heterogeneity has been obtained (ROBBINS et al. 1974).

Heterokaryons formed between fibroblasts from patients with X.p. and normal fibroblasts show, as expected, a restoration of repair. However also cells from different X.p. patients may complement each other; thus heterokaryons formed by fusion of repair-deficient fibroblasts from certain groups of X.p. patients showed an almost normal excision repair. So far five Complementation Groups have been distinguished designated A to E (KRAEMER et al. 1975; DE WEERD-KASTELEIN et al. 1972), and we can assume that at least five different genetic loci are involved.

Moreover, the observation that some patients which possess all the clinical symptoms of X.p. nevertheless appear capable of normal DNA excision repair had tempered the initial euphoria over the discovery of the molecular defect in DNA repair (CLEAVER 1973) until it was suggested that cells from X.p. variants (excision-proficient X.p.'s) are deficient in the postreplication repair (LEHMANN et al. 1975), and now a less severe defect in postreplication repair has been found in excision-defective X.p.'s in Complementation Groups A, B, C, and D (LEHMANN et al. 1977).

Taking into account these results we must ask what relationships exist between DNA damage, the operation of repair systems, mutagenesis, and carcinogenesis. In respect to the mutagenic process it is clear that ultimately the DNA is affected, but is this true for carcinogenesis? Although the correlation between mutagenic and oncogenic activity of *ultimate* carcinogens is a good one, the detailed molecular mechanism is not necessarily clear.

In microorganisms the concept of "error-prone" and "error-free" repair was put forward (WITKIN 1969, 1973, 1975, 1976). Excision-repair systems appear to be error-free, postreplication repair systems error-prone. Mutant organisms lacking excision repair will survive damage by means of the postreplication repair system and carry many induced mutations. Mutants lacking postreplication repair will survive by means of excision repair and will carry few induced mutations. Thus the concept of error-proneness, as it relates to mutagenesis and carcinogenesis, needs to be considered in relation to the known major repair processes in human cells (CLEAVER 1975). It is not known whether DNA damage initiates the induction of an SOS-like cluster of functions, including an error-prone repair activity in eukaryotic cells. But some effective SOS inducers are known to be carcinogenic in mammalian cells (GOZE et al. 1975). Mutagenic DNA polymerases which promote misincorporation of wrong bases in vitro in assays using synthetic templateprimers have been found in human cancer cells by SPRINGGATE and LOEB (1973). The enzyme TDT which polymerizes DNA by random "end-addition" without template instruction has also been detected in human leukemic cells (COLEMAN et al. 1974; MCCAFFREY et al. 1973; SRIVASTAVA and MINOWADA 1973).

The observation that both extracts of human leukemic lymphocytes and a purified DNA polymerase from avian myeloblastosis virus have exceptionally high error rates induced a hypothesis that relates mistakes in DNA replication as promoted by error-prone DNA-polymerases to tumor progression (LOEB et al. 1974).

The basic idea was that malignant changes result from random mutations producing defective polymerases. The finding of these workers that a DNA polymerase from an animal tumour virus is error-prone suggests the possibility that oncogenic viruses cause random mutation in this manner. They are proposing that infidelity of DNA replication may be responsible for tumour oncogenesis and progression and that this infidelity may be brought about by the introduction of error-prone viral polymerases into cells or by mutations in genes coding for cellular polymerases. The idea that errors in DNA replication may be important factors in initiation of malignant transformation have been proposed by some other workers (NELSON and MASON 1972; SARIN and GALLO 1974; SARASIN and MEUNIER-ROTIVAL 1976). Taking into account the present knowledge it seems possible to summarize the different speculations and hypothesis in the following simple figure.

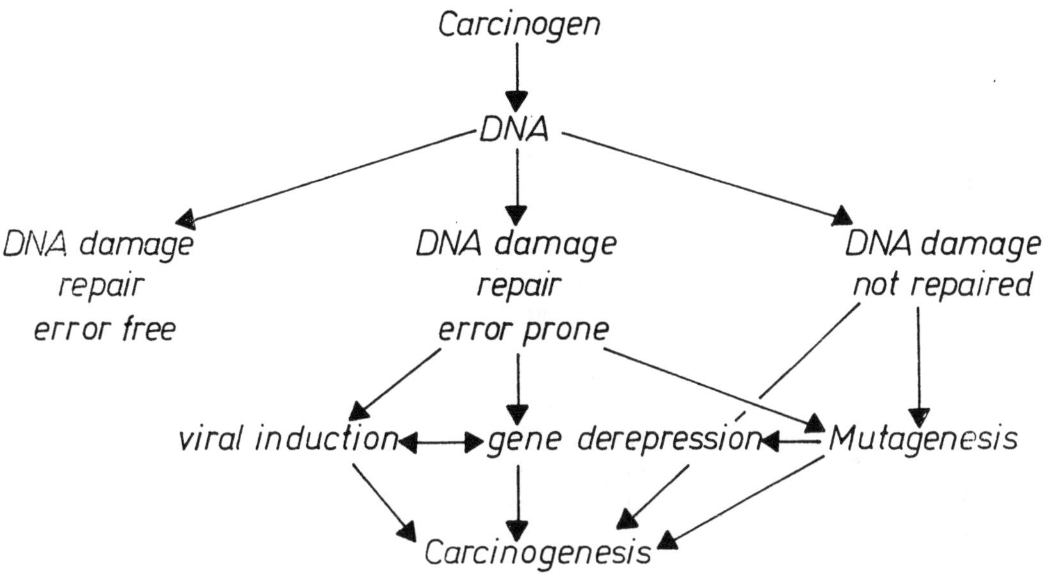

Fig. 1. Mechanisms for Carcinogenesis.

Another aspect of DNA repair in cancer research is the possibility to use the amount of excision repair as measure for screening carcinogenic substances (STICH et al. 1972) and for detecting organotropic actions of chemical carcinogens (STICH and KIESER 1974; LAISHES et al. 1975). Progress and problems using DNA repair to detect mutagens and carcinogens were reported by LIEBERMAN (1975) and DULBECCO (1977). The carcinogen-induced DNA repair in primary rat liver cell cultures was demonstrated as a possible screen for chemical carcinogens by G. M. WILLIAMS (1976), the role of DNA repair in the enhancement of viral transformation by chemical carcinogens was demonstrated by CASTO et al. (1976). The most sensitive method for detecting potential carcinogens has now been reported by WOLFF et al. (1977) analysing sister chromatid exchange induced by mutagenic carcinogens in normal and X.p. cells.
Irrespective of the question of carcinogenesis, a more profound understanding of the process of DNA repair may be important in the development of cancer treatment by

radiation and cytostatic substances. An impressive mass of evidence now supports the hypothesis that the lethal effect of ionizing radiations on cells is mediated by radiochemical damage induced in cellular DNA (KAPLAN 1974).
Lethality is known to be influenced by at least five interacting factors:

first, the nature and quality of the radiation,
second, the intrinsic radiation sensitivity of the DNA target,
third, the presence of dose modifying agents at the time of irradiation,
fourth, the ability of the cells to repair DNA damage, and
fifth, the influence of chemical, physiologic and genetic factors on these repair processes.

Taking into account the mentioned factors it would be desirable to answer two questions:

first, is it possible to find out different activities in DNA repair in tumour and normal cells, which would enable the therapist to tailor the treatment of cancer in relation to radiation dose, fractionation or selection of cytostatic drugs, and, second, is it possible to improve the radiation treatment of tumours by application of specific inhibitors of DNA repair processes in the cancer cells?

Trying to answer the first question we do not find encouraging results using alkaline sedimentation analysis. Comparing the sedimentation profiles of different cells from embryonic and malignant origin it was not possible to find significant differences in the repair capacity between cancer and normal cells after irradiation (MAGDON and SCHRÖDER 1971; 1972a, b).
The second question is extensively reviewed in this volume in the report "Studies on Alterations of DNA Processes" by SCHRÖDER and MAGDON and we may follow the idea that inhibition of repair of radiation induced DNA damage contributes significantly to the treatment-failure rate after radiotherapy for human cancer (BYFIELD 1974). Since tumour-cell number is a variable independent of the cell numbers which constitute the normal tissues in any given treatment volume, inhibition of the repair of X-ray-induced DNA damage in tumour cells is of increasing theoretical advantage during radiotherapy for advanced cancers, particularly for those of the epidermoid-transitional cell group in which the cure rate and the local control rate are closely related.
It is obvious that a continued search for chemical agents which inhibit repair in the postirradiation period is mandatory. If such agents can be identified, showing the required properties of low toxicity and differential entry into neoplastic cells, they could be expected to have a possibility to improve the therapy of human cancer.

References

[1] BOOTSMA, D., M. P. MULDER, F. POT, and J. A. COHEN: Mutation Res. **9**, 507–516 (1970)
[2] BOYCE, R. P., and P. HOWARD-FLANDERS: Proc. Nat. Acad. Sci. **51**, 293–300 (1964)
[3] BURK, P. G., M. A. LUTZNER, D. D. CLARK, and J. H. ROBBINS: J. Lab. Clin. Med. **77**, 759 (1971a)
[4] BURK, P. G., S. H. YUSPA, M. A. LUTZNER, and J. H. ROBBINS: Lancet **1**, 601 (1971b)
[5] BYFIELD, J. E.: Cancer Chemotherapy Reports, Part 1 **58**, 527–538 (1974)

[6] Casto, B. C., W. J. Pieczynski, N. Janosko, and J. A. DiPaolo: Chem.-Biol. Interactions **13**, 105—125 (1976)
[7] Cleaver, J. E.: Nature **218**, 652—656 (1968)
[8] Cleaver, J. E.: Proc. Nat. Acad. Sci. **63**, 428—435 (1969)
[9] Cleaver, J. E.: J. invest. Derm. **54**, 181 (1970a)
[10] Cleaver, J. E.: Int. J. Radiat. Biol. **18**, 557 (1970b)
[11] Cleaver, J. E.: J. invest. Derm. **58**, 124—128 (1972)
[12] Cleaver, J. E.: Cancer Res. **33**, 362 (1973)
[13] Cleaver, J. E.: J. invest. Derm. **60**, 374—380 (1973)
[14] Cleaver, J. E.: In: Methods in Cancer Research. Ed. by H. Busch, Vol. XI, New York, San Francisco, London: Academic Press 1975, pp. 123—165
[15] Coleman, M. S., J. J. Hutton, P. DeSimone, and F. J. Bollum: Proc. Nat. Acad. Sci. **71**, 4404—4408 (1974)
[16] De Weerd-Kastelein, E. A., W. J. Keijzer, and D. Bootsma: Nature New Biol. **238**, 80 (1972)
[17] Dulbecco, R.: Proc. R. Soc. Lond. B **196**, 117—130 (1977)
[18] Goze, A., A. Sarasin, Y. Moulé, and R. Devoret: Mutation Res. **28**, 1—7 (1975)
[19] Haddow, A.: Proc. roy. Soc. Med. **64**, 323—328 (1971)
[20] Kaplan, H. S.: In: Advances in Chemical Radiosensitization, International Atomic Energy Agency, Vienna, 1974, pp. 123—142
[21] Kraemer, K. H., H. G. Coon, R. A. Petingea, S. F. Barrett, A. E. Rahe, and J. H. Robbins: Proc. Nat. Acad. Sci. **72**, 59 (1975)
[22] Laishes, B. A., D. J. Koropatnick, and H. F. Stich: Proc. Soc. exp. Biol. Med. **149**, 978—982 (1975)
[23] Lehmann, A. R., S. Kirk-Bell, C. F. Arlett, M. C. Paterson, P. H. M. Lohman, E. A. De Weerd-Kastelein, and D. Bootsma: Proc. Nat. Acad. Sci. **72**, 219 (1975)
[24] Lehmann, A. R., S. Kirk-Bell, C. F. Arlett, S. A. Harcourt, E. A. De Weerd-Kastelein, W. Keijzer, P. Hall-Smith: Cancer Res. **37**, 904—910 (1977)
[25] Lett, J. T., I. Caldwell, C. J. Dean, and P. Alexander: Nature **214**, 790—792 (1967)
[26] Lieberman, M. W.: Ann. New York Acad. Sci. **269**, 37—42 (1975)
[27] Loeb, L. A., C. F. Springgate, and N. Battula: Cancer Res. **34**, 2311 (1974)
[28] Magdon, E., and E. Schröder: Strahlentherapie **142**, 195—200 (1971)
[29] Magdon, E., and H. Gummel: Dtsch. Gesundheitswes. **27**, 385—397 (1972)
[30] Magdon, E., and E. Schröder: Untersuchungen zur intrazellulären Reparatur von DNS-Einstrangbrüchen an Säugerzellen. Vortrag, Symposium Strahlenforschung der Gesellschaft für reine und angewandte Biophysik der DDR, Luisenthal, 17.—22. 4. 1972
[31] Magdon, E., and E. Schröder: Studia biophys. **30**, 162—163 (1972b)
[32] McCaffrey, R., D. F. Smoler, and D. Baltimore: Proc. Nat. Acad. Sci. **70**, 521—525 (1973)
[33] McGrath, R. A., and R. W. Williams: Nature **212**, 534—535 (1966)
[34] Nelson, R. L., and H. S. Mason: J. Theoret. Biol. **37**, 197—200 (1972)
[35] Pettijohn, D., and P. Hanawalt: J. Mol. Biol. **9**, 395—410 (1964)
[36] Rasmussen, R. E., and R. B. Painter: Nature **203**, 1360—1362 (1964)
[37] Robbins, J. H., K. H. Kraemer, M. A. Lutzner, B. W. Festoff, and H. G. Coon: Ann. Intern. Med. **80**, 221 (1974)
[38] Sarasin, A., and M. Meunier-Rotival: Biomedicine **24**, 306—316 (1976)
[39] Sarin, P. S., and R. C. Gallo: J. Biol. Chem. **249**, 8051—8053 (1974)
[40] Setlow, R. B., and W. L. Carrier: Proc. Nat. Acad. Sci. **51**, 226—231 (1964)
[41] Setlow, R. B.: Radiat. Res. Suppl. **6**, 220—226 (1966)
[42] Setlow, R. B., J. D. Regan, J. German, and W. L. Carrier: Proc. Nat. Acad. Sci. **64**, 1035—1041 (1969)
[43] Springgate, C., and L. A. Loeb: Proc. Nat. Acad. Sci. **70**, 245—249 (1973)

[44] Srivastava, B. I. S., and J. Minowada: Biochem. Biophys. Res. Commun. **51**, 529–535 (1973)
[45] Stich, H. F., R. H. C. San, J. A. Miller, and E. C. Miller: Nature New Biol. **238**, 9–10 (1972)
[46] Stich, H. F., and D. Kieser: Proc. Soc. exp. Biol. Med. **145**, 1339 (1974)
[47] Strauss, B. S.: Life Sci. **15**, 1685 (1975)
[48] Williams, G. M.: Cancer Letters **1**, 231–236 (1976)
[49] Witkin, E. M.: Ann. Rev. Genet. **3**, 525 (1969)
[50] Witkin, E. M.: An. Acad. Bras. Cienc., Suppl. **45**, 188–192 (1973)
[51] Witkin, E. M.: Genetics Suppl. **79**, 199–213 (1975)
[52] Witkin, E. M.: Bacteriol. Rev. **40**, 869–907 (1976)
[53] Wolff, S., B. Rodin, and J. E. Cleaver: Nature **265**, 347–349 (1977)

FUNDAMENTALS OF DNA REPAIR

Single and Double Strand Breaks in the Cellular DNA

V. Drášil and V. Jurášková

Institute of Biophysics, Czechoslovac Academy of Sciences, Brno

The isokinetic centrifugation of DNA in alkaline and neutral sucrose density gradient was introduced into molecular biological research approximately 13 years ago [1]. As shown by the wide development of this method in later years, the changes in the molecular weight of DNA following relatively low doses of ionizing radiation or the action of other agents of a physical or chemical nature, may be investigated in this way. Centrifugation of DNA in density gradients makes it possible to study induction and elimination of single and double strand breaks in cellular DNA, and thus it proves indispensable in the study of repair processes. At the same time it has been shown that even the DNA complexes with other cell components, for instance with membranes, may be investigated by this method. The use of centrifugation in density gradients thus has a wide application. This contribution is focussed predominantly on problems of single and double breaks in cellular DNA. As the results and interpretations are closely dependent on the ultracentrifugal technique used, considerable attention is devoted here to experience of a methodical character.

I. Isokinetic centrifugation of DNA

On centrifugation, a macromolecule in aqueous or other medium is influenced by a force which makes it move in a radial direction and by friction inhibiting such a movement. The first force (P) may be expressed $P = m'\omega^2 r$, where m' designates a particle's weight diminished by bouyant force, ω stands for angular speed and r represents the radius of rotation. According to the character of the medium, the m' value may be positive, zero, or negative.

The friction (f) which inhibits the movement of a particle in solution depends on the size and form of such a particle, and further, it is a function of the velocity of its movement ($f = F/v/$). If a macromolecule's motion is followed along a very short path (ds), then it may be observed that, in motion, the friction value increases so that it compensates action of centrifugal force; along such short path a particle moves with constant velocity. Hence, it is valid that the ratio between particle's velocity (v) and centrifugal acceleration at a given point is constant.

$$\frac{v}{\omega^2 r} = k \qquad v = \omega^2 r \cdot t$$

The constant k is expressed in time units, $k = 10^{-13}$ sec $= 1S$. If the quality of the medium in which the motion of a particle occurs is constant, then the particle's veloc-

ity should gradually increase because the value of acceleration ($\omega^2 r$) increases proportionally to the rotation radius accordingly to the distance from the rotation axis. However, the sedimentation constant (for H_2O usually given at 20 °C) may be influenced by changes of density and viscosity of the medium.
For such a case, it is valid that

$$S_{t,m} = S_{20,w} \frac{1 - \bar{v}\varrho_{t,m}\eta_{20,w}}{1 - \bar{v}\varrho_{20,w}\eta_{t,m}}$$

where $\bar{v}$ is the partial specific volume, $\eta_{t,m}$ is the viscosity of the medium and $\varrho_{t,m}$ is its density.
It was demonstrated by HERSHEY and BURGI with centrifugation of DNA in 5—20% sucrose gradients [2] that increased density and viscosity of the medium nearly completely compensated the increase of centrifugal acceleration with increasing radius; the movement of DNA in such a gradient is linear. This is valid predominantly for case of centrifugation carried out in the ultracentrifuge Spinco SL 50 with swing out rotor 3×5 ml.
Isokinetic centrifugation exhibits a lot of advantages, mainly concerning the calculation of the sedimentation constant from the path at which a particle travels during centrifugation, and further, concerning calibration of the gradient by means of DNA of known S — value, or of known molecular weight.
Naturally, in the case of different type of centrifuge it need not be valid that 5—20% sucrose density gradient occurs with a linear dependence between the duration of centrifugation and the pathway along which the DNA travels from the surface of the gradient. For a swing-out rotor 3×5 ml of JANETZKI VAC 60 and 601 ultracentrifuge types (which exhibit lower r than the Spinco), we found that at the beginning of centrifugation velocity increases approximately to a distance of 2 cm from the surface and then linear movement occurs between this distance and the bottom of the tube [3].
As shown above, the determination of the sedimentation constant in a preparative ultracentrifuge is a relatively complex problem and the resulting values may often contain considerable error, which, in our experience, may be as high as 10%. To maintain this error below the value mentioned, it is essential to keep constant conditions for gradient preparation and its distribution into individual fractions after centrifugation. For the time being, for linear density gradient preparations, a continual mixing of both solutions representing the upper and lower concentration limits in the mixer and slow influx into the centrifugation tube is strongly recommended. It seems that it is not conclusive whether layers begin to form at the highest concentration and rise work upwards, or whether a mixed solution is supplied permanently at the bottom of the tube with increasing concentration. In the latter case, components of lower concentration are gradually lifted.
On gradient distribution into individual fractions, it is necessary to adopt a method with which constant fraction volume is ensured. In this sense, drop-counting is not satisfactory because — due to the different composition of solution in the tube and due to the detergents with which cells are lysed — the size of the drops varies. As far as detergents are concerned, some of them precipitate in a medium containing more than 2—3% sucrose. A precipitate sediments forming a ring approximately 1/3 of the way from the surface, and may thus damage the sample tested.
A layer of material placed at the top of the gradient is not infinitely thin. To measure

the DNA pathway from the surface, it is advisable to determine its starting point. If a linear movement through whole gradient is assumed, the starting point may be determined graphically, using the peak movement records at several time intervals. Starting point is obtained by extrapolation of the peak position for zero-time of centrifugation.

II. Determination of molecular weight of DNA in the preparative ultracentrifuge

The calculation of the molecular weight of DNA results from its sedimentation constant $S_{20,w}$ and the empirical relationship between sedimentation constant and molecular weight. This relation is usually given as the $S_{20,w} = kM^{\alpha}$ type of equation. The values k and α depend on whether the DNA is linear or circular, native or denatured, centrifuged at neutral or alkaline pH etc. Numerous equations obtained by means of DNA of known molecular weight may be found in the literature. We may point out that the values k and α gradually become more precise. Most of today's empirical relationships were obtained by means of DNA isolated from viruses and bacteriophages where extreme high molecular weight reaches approximately 1.3×10^8 D. The possibility of using the equation obtained in this manner even in the case of a molecular weight of the order 10^9 is discussed by numerous authors. Such equations are then carefully employed in most of the contributions. However, some theoretical studies of recent years indicate that it will be possible in the future to derive such relations from fundamental physicochemical properties of the DNA macromolecule [4, 5].

In the case of isokinetic centrifugation, $S_{20,w} = Cd$ (d distance of the material from starting point of sedimentation). Thus, if two kinds of DNA exhibiting sedimentation coefficients S_1 and S_2 are given, we may write

$$S_1 = Cd_1 = kM_1^{\alpha}$$

$$S_2 = Cd_2 = kM_2^{\alpha}$$

so that

$$\frac{d_1}{d_2} = \left(\frac{M_1}{M_2}\right)^{\alpha}$$

With this method, a gradient may be calibrated if at least one molecular weight value is known with sufficient accuracy. For a centrifuge Spinco (SW rotor 50) equations of the following type are often employed for the calculation of molecular weight of i-th fraction (6).

$$M_i = k\left(\frac{d_i}{\omega^2 t}\right)^{\alpha}$$

k constant
d distance from gradient surface
t centrifugation time given in hrs.

III. Determination of number of breaks in DNA

Calculating the number of breaks induced in the DNA macromolecule, we may start with the equation:

$$N = \frac{M_0}{M_1} - 1$$

N number of breaks, M_0 original molecular weight, M_1 final molecular weight

In practice, experiments bring a more complex situation because a wide set of DNA molecules, differing in molecular weight, is induced in the system. Such a heterogenous system may be obtained by the action of radiation, or by the action of another factor. With gradual polymer fracture, it is valid that with an increasing number of breaks (higher than 5 for a macromolecule) the fragments show random distribution of molecular weights [7]. Then, in the equation mentioned above, molecular weights are substituted by the M_n value calculated from the relationship:

$$M_n = \frac{\sum w_i}{\sum w_i/M_i}$$

w_i total mass of the DNA of i-th fraction
M_i molecular weight of i-th fraction

For centrifugation of DNA in density gradients, M_n-values may be established by various methods. The most simple one is to start at average molecular weights of individual fractions which are introduced into this equation. Radioactivity of the fractions which represents a quantity being firmly related to total DNA mass of the fraction ($w_i = kA_i$) is substituted for w_i-value. In the first fractions at the meniscus radioactivity is bound to small molecules and therefore even its low values represent a great number of molecules; it may substantially depress the final M_n-values. Further, in this gradient range there often remain low molecular precursors which are not quantitatively removed while preparing the gradient for radioactive measurement. For this reason, calculation of M_n-value in the above manner is accurate only for the case where the peak of radioactivity distribution occurs at the centre of the gradient and where the first fractions (approximately 10—15% of total number of fractions) do not contain an increased level of radioactivity. Many authors do not include such initial fractions into the calculation.

The theoretical calculations mentioned above [7] indicate that $M_w = 2M_n$.

$$M_w = \frac{\sum w_i M_i}{\sum w_i}$$

As is apparent from this equation, M_w is less sensitive to the presence of small molecules at the beginning of the gradient. Therefore some authors base their calculation on M_w and evidently use $M_n = \frac{M_w}{2}$. However, analysis of the results demonstrates that such a relation is not always real. The M_w-value is sensitive to the incidence of individual large molecules at gradient's end. But fast sedimenting DNA complexes may also be present here, and thus even in this case it is necessary to make careful calculations and include, if possible, only data which really belong to the fundamental set of molecular weights of DNA.

Another method of determining the M_n-value, which can also serve as a control of whether distribution of DNA molecular weights in the gradient corresponds to theoretical assumptions, was reported by DEAN et al. [8]. For such a case, we use $\log C/M_i \times \Delta M_i$ plotted versus M_i. (C radioactivity of i-th fraction of the gradient, M_i molecular weight of DNA in the fraction, ΔM_i range of molecular weights in i-th fraction.) If molecular weight distribution is in agreement with theory, then a graphical plotting of the above relationship gives a straight line of $-1/M_n$ slope.

The above indicates the fact that the distribution of DNA molecular weights in the gradient has to approximate to the values derived from theory on the cleavage of linear macromolecules. On the basis of today's experience in many laboratories, it may be stated that the lower the M_n-values exhibited by the centrifuged DNA, the easier it is to achieve the above condition. In the course of sedimentation, individual DNA macromolecules have to behave as independent particles. Hence it follows that a low DNA concentration is required in the solution, and further, it is abvious that even other cell components which remain in spite of detergents and the action of high pH bound to DNA may give unfavourable response. A rapid and relatively authentic test of whether the DNA centrifuged corresponds roughly to these criteria, is the influence of the rotor's revolutions on the $S_{20,w}$ value. If the $S_{20,w}$ value rises with increasing $\omega^2 r$, it is not possible to make appropriate conclusions on molecular weight because sedimentation does not apparently occur under the above conditions.

The method of calculation of molecular weights and numbers of breaks occuring in the molecule using radioactivity distribution in the gradient so far reported can be used everywhere. But the results have to be interpreted carefully because not all the sources of error can be estimated even by detailed treatment. Higher accuracy of calculations and results may be achieved by the use of a computer. Some reports published recently [9, 10] point out to a certain possibility of computerization in this field. New methods of analysis of molecular weight distribution in the gradient by means of a computer make possible better evaluation of some than previously. This refers mainly to the centrifugation of DNA isolated from non-irradiated cells and exhibiting a molecular weight higher than 10^8 Dalton.

To conclude this section dealing with methods of molecular weight determination for DNA and its changes by means of centrifugation in density gradients, we may state: from the qualitative point of view, this technique offers valuable information. As demonstrated by the shift of the peak radioactivity in the gradient, molecular weight alterations are often immediately evident. With this approach, for instance, the presence or absence of the system of repairing breaks in the DNA macromolecule after induction by various factors, may easily be proved. On the other hand, quantitative evaluation should be considered with reservation especially when comparing results obtained in different laboratories. For such purpose further progress which might lead to an increase in the reliability of the techniques used, even in the quantitative aspect, is required.

IV. Sedimentation of DNA from non-irradiated cells

The molecular weight of the DNA of bacterial cell chromosome reaches up to 10^9 Dalton value. The molecular weight of the DNA of mammalian cell chromosome would approximate a 10^{11} Dalton value, if only one macromolecule is present in the chromosome.

Linear macromolecules corresponding to such molecular weight may be in the range of mm—size up to cm—size. Centrifugation of DNA of such dimensions exhibits a certain abnormality compared with material of molecular weight lowered by one or more orders.

Sedimentation constants of material prepared by short lysis of mammalian cells at the gradient's surface (up to 60 min) reach several hundreds S. In the case of alkaline gradient, that value is as high as $800S$, if mammalian cells are lysed for only 20 min. In the case of neutral gradient treated under identical conditions, material with a sedimentation constant of up to $400S$ is obtained. Rapidly sedimenting material which exhibits a sedimentation constant higher than $100S$ is attained even after lysis of bacterial cells.

Data on the sedimentation constant of DNA both of unirradiated animal and bacterial cells are of importance only as an indicator that the material sediments rapidly. In that case, "sedimentation constant" is not in fact a constant because its value depends on acceleration $\omega^2 r$ under which centrifugation is carried out. With increasing $\omega^2 r$, even distribution of activity in the gradient is changed, the peak becomes so narrow that most activity is found in 2—3 fractions. Density of the rapidly sedimenting component in CsCl gradients was studied and determined to be significantly below 1.7. Thus it is obvious that, in that case, it is not free DNA, but a complex of DNA with other cell components [11]. It seems that it is not a matter of protein—complex, but of substances of lipoid character. Perhaps it is the matter of DNA which remains connected, even after cellular lysis, with nuclear membranes or with material which constitutes the chromosomal skeleton of mammalian cell [12].

Lysis of animal cells in alkaline medium ought to lead to release of denatured DNA. However, a certain time-period is necessary to separate both the complementary strands. The duration depends on the square of molecular weight of the DNA, as was proved by Davison for some kinds of DNA of molecular weight up to 1.3×10^8 Dalton [13]. Extrapolating data of molecular weight of DNA at 10^9, we may read a time of 20 min necessary for the lysis. If DNA of molecular weight 10^{10} is taken into account, then the time essential for strand separation is more than 33 hrs. It is probable that on short lysis of mammalian cells in alkaline gradient, a great portion of DNA remains in the native state. When observing dependence of sedimentation constant on duration of the lysis at mammalian cells [14], it is demonstrated that after approximately 9 hrs., sedimentation constant is fixed at nearly $167S$-value; if Studier's equation for molecular weight calculation is used [15], value of 5.6×10^8 Dalton is obtained. A DNA of such molecular weight is then considered to be a sub-unit of the nucleic acid of a mammalian chromosome [16, 17].

Reviewing results on centrifugation of DNA from non-irradiated cells of predominantly mammalian origin as obtained to date, it may be assumed that a higher accuracy should be required anyway. For instance, there is no clear answer on what structural arrangement large DNA macromolecules have in solution after lysis. Simultaneous centrifugation of DNAs labelled with ^{14}C and ^{3}H indicates that no entanglement of the macromolecules probably takes place. Hence it seems that the DNA forms multiple "superhelices" with certain analogous properties to the circular DNA of some phages, viruses or cellular organelles. With regard to its shape, sedimentation constant of such DNA is substantially higher than that of linear molecule of the same size [5].

V. Induction of single and double strand breaks in cellular DNA by ionizing radiation

The lowest doses of ionizing radiation which are reflected in a change of sedimentation velocity of the DNA are in the range of irradiation of the cells between 100—200 rad [18]. After irradiation of mammalian cells with this dose, a decrease of the sedimentation constant of the DNA containing complex occurs on centrifugation both in neutral and alkaline sucrose gradients. With an increasing radiation dose a sharp decrease in sedimentation constant appears at the beginning, then, a gradual lowering of the sharp peak of activity may be observed. Molecular weight distribution in the gradient gradually becomes a slope which approximates to the theoretical distribution of molecular weight. This is apparently manifested with the case of alkaline gradient where the DNA is freed from a complex (or its total denaturation takes place) due to high pH even after doses of a few krad. Release of DNA from a complex with other components due to irradiation is slower, if a neutral gradient is used. For the occurrence of most of the DNA in the form of "free" DNA in the gradient, the doses should be 20 krad or higher [12, 17]. Free DNA is characterized by density of about 1.7 and further by molecular weight distribution in the gradient corresponding to the presumptions given above. Achievement of free-DNA in the gradient is of great importance for accurate calculation both of molecular weight and the number of breaks. But this feature has an important role even in a qualitative comparison of radiation effects made on the basis of activity-peak in the gradient. It was illustrated by a more detailed study of the effect of doses in the range from 100 rad to 15 krad on the sedimentation of material containing DNA after lysis of mammalian cells that, at first, in neutral gradient the sedimentation constant decreased from 400 to 80 S after a dose which reached 2500 rad. On a further increase of dose, a slight increase (up to 120 S) occurred when the dose reached the range 8000 to 10000 rad. Beginning at this point, a further decrease takes place with the rise in dose (author's unpublished results). For case of sedimentation constant increase between 2500—8000 rad, gradual release of DNA from the complex and a increase of density of centrifuged material may be considered. But these results illustrate that quantitative evaluation of radiation effect by means of neutral gradient is hardly possible in the given range of doses. Even on qualitative evaluation, incorrect interpretation may be made with respect to abnormal behaviour of centrifuged material.

Beginning with a few krad level of doses, the number of single breaks in cellular DNA is a linear function of dose. This dependence may be demonstrated by plotting inverse molecular weight value ($1/M_n$) against dose. Hence linear dependence may be assumed even for doses between 0 and 2500 rad. Extrapolating a straight line illustrating dependence of $1/M_n$-value on dose into the zero-dose region leads us to the findings that such a straight-line intersects the y-axis at the point where the $1/M_n$-value appears to be 10^{-10} or lower. Such interpolation indicates that in chromosomes the DNA forms only one unit of molecular weight of 10^{10} Dalton, or that the number of sub-units is low [19, 20].

Induction of single breaks in cellular DNA by ionizing radiation was studied in very different types of cells. As presented in many contributions, sensitivity of DNA is expressed either in energy units which should be absorbed by one break formation (eV/break), or in the number of breaks calculated for a unit of dose. Reviewing the results of numerous reports, it may be noted that sensitivity of DNA to induction of single breaks in various cell types varies with unremarkable deviations. For many types of cells 40—70 eV

(Tab. 1) is required for single break formation. Making calculations aimed at higher accuracy, we are led sometimes to additional corrections, but it is stated that from this point of view, sensitivity of cellular DNA approximates to that of dry DNA, of which it is known that about 56 *eV* corresponds to 1 single break [36]. Such a comparison may give rise to the assumption that on break formation in the DNA in vivio, the direct action of radiation is mainly involved; here is meant ionization and excitation in the macromolecule. But as follows from Tab. 1, deviations of individual values are high enough to include even a certain ratio of indirect radiation effect on break formation. Another conclusion which may be read into Tab. 1 is that there is no dependence between radiosensitivity of the cell and sensitivity of this DNA to single break induction. Exceptional case is a cell of *Micrococcus radiodurans* where a significant percentage of cell population survives doses as high as several hundred thousand rad, on the other hand, there is a mammalian cell of D_0 at 100 rad level. For both cases, about 50— 70 *eV* absorbed energy is needed for single break induction in the DNA.

Table 1. DNA single and double breaks in various organisms.

Organism	Conditions of irradiation	*eV*/break		References
		single	double	
T4 and T7 phage	O_2	71	1250	21
	N_2	110	2500	
T7 phage	10^{-3} M histidine	69	390	22
T1 phage	10^{-1} M histidine	86	1730	23
T7 phage	N_2	42	530	24
phage	O_2	75	—	25
in *E. coli* K12	N_2	210	—	
E. coli	air	333	—	1
E. coli	O_2	91	—	26
E. coli	O_2	75	—	27
M. radiodurans	O_2 ± EDTA	50	—	28
	N_2 + EDTA	50	—	
	N_2	150	—	
M. radiodurans	air	50	1060	29
	N_2	140	500	
M. radiodurans	O_2	40	520	30
Acholeplasma	O_2	58	469	31
laidlawii A	N_2	158	1862	
L5178Y	O_2	66	—	29
cells	N_2	66	—	
L5178Y	air	70	—	20
cells	N_2	150	—	
L5178Y cells	air	—	2900	19
Ehrlich ascites cells	air	280	—	32
Chinese hamster cells	air	116	—	6
Chinese hamster cells	air	—	600	33
Chinese hamster cells	air	82,6	—	35
	N_2	284	—	
Rat thymocytes	air, 10M eV electrons	109	1940	34

The yield of DNA single-strand breaks induced by irradiation is affected by many factors. Several authors have observed that the presence of oxygen during irradiation does not change the number of breaks but affects the possibility of their repair, mainly by means of ligase [8, 37]. Most recent reports in which number of breaks was studied immediately after pulse irradiation (lasting for only a few milisec.) illustrate that O_2 presence may lead to approximately 3-times higher production of breaks than the irradiation performed under oxygen-free atmosphere [38, 39].
The radiation yield of breaks is further lowered by protective substances [21, 40, 41] or by changes in the physical conditions of irradiation (irradiation carried out at −74 or −196 °C) [42]. Oxygen effect, and the effect of other factors on single break induction shows that — beside direct radiation action — indirect action is also involved. In our opinion, the indirect radiation effect is at least equal to that of direct action.
Simultaneously with single break production there are double breaks induced in cellular DNA, formed according to two, possible mechanisms: a double break arises as a single event when opposite strands of DNA at a distance of less than several nucleotide pairs are broken. If sparsely ionizing radiation is used, this process is significantly less probable than that of single break formation. Another mechanism producing double breaks is based on the gradual occurrence of two single breaks sufficiently close in opposite DNA strands. In the first case, the number of double breaks increases linearly with dose, in the latter case, number of breaks depends on the square of dose. Experimental results show [19, 34, 43] that dependence of the number of double breaks is linear with respect to dose. Thus, it may be assumed that most of them are induced by the first mechanism mentioned above.
Data on the energy rate essential for 1 double break are summarized also in Tab. 1. It is shown here that the values are at least 1 order higher than those for single breaks. Variations given by individual authors are higher than in the case of single strand breaks. One of the unfavourable factors is probably the magnitude of dose necessary for cell irradiation resulting in the possibility of evaluating quantitatively the results of DNA centrifugation in neutral gradient. The tens of krads necessary are beyond the threshold where a cell might survive and thus we do not exclude that at such high doses, lesions of other cell structures secondarily affecting the course of damage to DNA may occur.
To conclude this part of the contribution we would like to point out a feature which — in our opinion — is not sufficiently studied: it is an initial sharp decrease of sedimentation constant in the neutral gradient which takes place after irradiation of the cell with a dose of 100 rad or more. For instance, if molecular weight of DNA is presumed to be 5×10^{10} Dalton, then a 100 rad dose leads to absorption of approximately 500 eV sufficient to induce about 10 single breaks. Their average distance measures about 5×10^9 Dalton. In spite of the low number of breaks and their wide separation remarkable change of sedimentation occurs. Future studies ought to discover what a structure of DNA may be the basis for these changes.

VI. Repair of breaks in cellular DNA after irradiation

The technique used for the investigation of alterations in molecular weight of cell DNA by means of centrifugation in density gradients makes it possible to discover not only breaks induced by radiation, but enables us also to answer the question of the further fate of the DNA damaged by radiation. It is clearly evidenced by many contributions dealing with that problem that single breaks are promptly repaired in the cell. Repair is reflected in an increase both of molecular weight and of sedimentation constant of DNA which gradually reaches the values obtained from non-irradiated cells, e.g. a few hundreds *S*. The DNA in such a case again obtains the properties of the complex mentioned above. Repair of single breaks of DNA is one of the procedures which may be examined when the cells are at the most different stages of phylogenetic development, from bacteria to mammalian cell. This process is probably of a complex character. Detailed investigation indicates that several enzymatic systems might be involved. It is not surprising that the conception of single break includes a few types of break in DNA strands differing in their free ends. Rejoining of the ends requires either their previous treatment, or the presence of special enzymatic systems (one or more) by means of which it is performed.

According to the rate and conditions under which repair occurs, some authors [37] distinguish ultrafast, fast and slow repair. The first one is probably realized by ligase, which connects breaks with $5'PO_4$ and $3'OH$ ends [44, 45]. Repair of this type lasts for a period shorter than one minute, even if the temperature is decreased to 0 °C. On longer irradiation of the cells ultrafast repair might misrepresent the yield of single breaks induced. Recently, in order to eliminate its influence, pulse irradiation and very rapid lysis of the cells [38] has been employed.

Incubation of irradiated cells at 37 °C leads to rapid repair which rejoins fragments of DNA by polymerase action. DNA synthesis is not essential for this process.

Incubation in cultivation medium at 37 °C prolonged to period of few hours leads to the repair of further breaks so that the total quantity of breaks repaired is about 90% or more. It is not easy to determine the amount of unrepaired breaks because the method does not allow the estimation of this with enough accuracy. Besides, even though we find a certain amount of the DNA (for instance 10%) in the gradient exhibiting low molecular weight even after incubation, it is not clear whether such DNA is randomly distributed in the cells, or whether it is the matter of total DNA of small group of the population studied.

The repair of single breaks in cellular DNA after irradiation is not one of the processes specifically induced by ionizing radiation. It seems that each cell has a mechanism which permanently controls and recovers integrity of its DNA. Enzymes which are a constituent part of such a system, are already present in the cells prior to irradiation and may start their activity immediately after break formation in a macromolecule. These enzymes repair even damage induced by factors of chemical nature [46]. Regarding the relationship to cell survival after irradiation, induction and repair of single breaks does not seem to be the factor responsible for the death of the cell. For instance, such a process may be eliminated by rapidly cooling the animal cells to −74 to −196 °C. In the first hours after thawing it is not possible to detect any repair of the DNA, within irradiated cells under incubation in cultivation medium, and a slight decrease of molecular weight of DNA in the cell is observed. However, more than 50% of the cells survive this treatment [42].

The repair of single breaks of DNA takes place in the cell even after irradiation with doses of about 10^5 rad. It was believed that a repair mechanism in the cell disposes with numerous sets of individual repair-enzymes so that even a high dose is not sufficient to inactivate them all. The question was also analysed in detail whether repair is per-

formed in another manner in the cases where irradiation is carried out in the absence of O_2. It was also pointed out that the difference between irradiation made in the presence or absence of oxygen may be found in the feature that — in the later case the breaks are better repaired [37]. But it seems that, as shown above, such a assumption is not well-founded. It was also a question take into account concerning the eventual relationship of single breaks in the DNA to the so-called repair of sub-lethal damage [50]. Comparing conditions under which both the types of repair function or are inactivated, it is recognized that it is not possible to make the repair of sub-lethal damage to the cell identical with that of single breaks in the DNA.
In contrast to single break repair, a double break repair according to today's results, seems to be a more complicated process. Some authors who dealt with that problem did not usually observe the repair of double breaks in mammalian cells [19, 47], where doses in the range from a few tens of thousands to 10^5 rad were used. Information collected by other laboratories indicates that, in certain cases, even double breaks may be repaired after irradiation [48, 51]. In *M. radiodurans* cells, repair of double breaks was fully evidenced [30]. In connection with double break repair, a relationship of double breaks to the cell survival after irradiation is often discussed. It is of interest to point out the hypothesis of Abel et al. [49]. who believe that the DNA of the chromosome is divided into sub-units of molecular weight of approximately 5×10^9 Dalton (750 subunits/cell.) Sub-unit ends are held by a structure which supports the skeleton of the chromosome. If one double break arises in a sub-unit, a repair may occur. Two breaks or more cause a lost of DNA section between them and thus it is a matter of lethal effect. According to the authors cited, the repair of a double break in a DNA sub-unit is identical with the repair of sub-lethal damage to the cell by radiation [50]. Most experimental data is in close agreement with that hypothesis. This hypothesis might also elucidate why after densely ionizing radiation no repair of sub-lethal damage occurs because in this case, numerous double breaks arise in close proximity.

VII. Conclusion

The study of the breaks induced in the molecule of cellular DNA radiation showed that the cell exhibited several mechanisms which were able to repair that damage. Such mechanisms repair even breaks which are induced by factors other than radiation. With a method originally developed for the study of radiation effects we succeeded, though only partly, in finding one of the general mechanisms which supports exact transfer of information by means of DNA.

References

[1] Mc Grath, R. A., Williams, R. W.: Nature **212**, 534 (1966)
[2] Burgi, E., Hershey, A. D.: Biophys. J. **3**, 309 (1963)
[3] Huťkova, J., Drášil, V.: Coll. Czechoslov. Chem. Comm. **37**, 1938 (1972)
[4] Reinert, K. E., Strassburger, J., Triebel, H.: Biopolymers **10**, 285 (1971)
[5] Böttger, M., Bierwolf, D., Wunderlich, V., Graffi, A.: Bioch. Biophys. Acta **232**, 21 (1971)
[6] Gillespie, C. J., Gislason, G. S., Dugle, D. L., Champan, J. D.: Rad. Res. **51**, 272 (1972)
[7] Charlesby, A.: Proc. R. Soc. A. **224**, 120 (1954)

[8] Dean, C. J., Ormerod, M. G., Serianni, K. W., Alexander, P.: Nature **222**, 1042 (1969)
[9] Ehmann, U. K., Lett, J. T.: Rad. Res. **54**, 152 (1973)
[10] Fox, R. A.: Int. J. Rad. Biol. **30**, 67 (1976)
[11] Ormerod, M. G., Lehmann, A. R.: Bioch. Biophys. Acta **247**, 369 (1971)
[12] Ormerod, M. G., Lehmann, A. R.: Bioch. Biophys. Acta **228**, 331 (1971)
[13] Davison, P. F.: J. Mol. Biol. **22**, 97 (1966)
[14] Klucis, E. S., Lett, J. T.: Analyt. Biochemistry **35**, 480 (1970)
[15] Studier, F. W.: J. Mol. Biol. **12**, 525 (1965)
[16] Lett, J. T., Klucis, E. S., Sun, C.: Biophys. J. **10**, 277 (1970)
[17] Elkind, M. M., Kamper, C.: Biophys. J. **10**, 237 (1970)
[18] Drášil, V., Karpfel, Z., Jurášková, V.: Peaceful uses of atomic energy IAEA, Vienna **13**, 381 (1972)
[19] Lehmann, A. R., Ormerod, M. G.: Biochim. Biophys. Acta **217**, 268 (1970)
[20] Lett, J. T., Caldwell, I. W. R., Dean, C. J., Alexander, P.: Nature **214**, 790 (1967)
[21] Schans, v. d. G. P., Blok, Y.: Int. J. Rad. Biol. **17**, 25 (1970)
[22] Freifelder, D.: Rad. Res. **29**, 329 (1966)
[23] Bohne, L., Coquerelle, T., Hagen, U.: Int. J. Rad. Biol. **3**, 205 (1970)
[24] Freifelder, D.: Proc. Natl. Ac. Sc. **54**, 128 (1965)
[25] Boyce, R. P., Tepper, M.: Virology **34**, 344 (1968)
[26] Freifelder, D.: J. Mol. Biol. **35**, 303 (1968)
[27] Town, C. D., Smith, K. C., Kaplan, H. S.: Science **172**, 851 (1971)
[28] Dean, C. J., Ormerod, M. G., Serianni, R. W., Alexander, P.: Nature **222**, 5198 (1969)
[29] Dean, C. J., Feldschreiber, P., Lett, J. T.: Nature **209**, 49 (1966)
[30] Burrel, A. D., Feldschreiber, P., Dean, C. J.: Biochim. Biophys. Acta **247**, 38 (1971)
[31] Huťkova, J., Drášil, V., Liška, B.: Zbl. Bakt. Abt. II., **130**, 424 (1975)
[32] Moroson H., Furean, M.,: Rad. Res. **44**, 713 (1970)
[33] Corry, P. M., Cole, A.: Rad. Res. **36**, 528 (1968)
[34] Coquerelle, T., Bopp, A., Kessler, B., Hagen, U.: Int. J. Rad. Biol. **24**, 397 (1973)
[35] Dugle, D. L., Chapman, J. D., Gillespie, C. J., Borsa, J., Nebb, R. G., Meeker, B. E., Reuvers, A. P.: Int. J. Rad. Biol. **22**, 545 (1972)
[36] Neary, G. J., Horgan V. J., Bance, D. A., Stretch, A.: Int. J. Rad. Biol. **22**, 525 (1972)
[37] Town, C. D., Smith, K. C., Kaplan, H. S.: Curr. Top. Radiat. Res., **8**, 351 (1973)
[38] Sapora, O., Fielden, E. M., Loverock, P. S.: Rad. Res. **64**, 431 (1975)
[39] Boye, E., Johanson, I., Brustad, T.,: J. Bacteriol. **119**, 522 (1974)
[40] Ginsberg, D. M., Webster, H. K.: Rad. Res. **39**, 421 (1969)
[41] Antoku, S.: Rad. Res. **65**, 130 (1976)
[42] Drášil V., Juraskoví V.: Studia Biophysica: **61**, 33 (1977)
[43] Veatch, W., Okada, S.: Biophys. J. **9**, 330 (1969)
[44] Gaziev, A. I., Sergeeva, S. A., Zakrevskaja, D. T.: Studia Biophys. **42**, 203 (1974)
[45] Jacobs, A., Bopp, A., Hagen, U.: Int. J. Rad. Biol. **22**, 431 (1972)
[46] Horikawa, M., Fukuhara, M., Suzuki, F., Nikaido, O., Sugahara, T.: Exp. Cell Res. **70**, 349 (1972)
[47] Horikawa, M., Nikaido, O., Tanaka, T., Nagata, H., Sugahara, T.: Exp. Cell Res. **63**, 325 (1970)
[48] Hartwig, M., Handschak, V., Rakow, A.: Abstracts of the First Radiobiological Conference of Socialist Countries, Bedřichov, ČSSR, 1974, p. 358
[49] Regel, K., Abel, H., Kampf, G.: in preparation
[50] Elkind, M. M., Sutton, H.: Rad. Res. **13**, 556 (1960)
[51] Tuschl, H., Klein, W., Kocsis, F., Kovac, R., Altmann, H.: Studia Biophys. **50**, 55 (1975)

Some Aspects of Unscheduled DNA synthesis in Irradiated Cells

L. Beneš, E. Magdon*, E. Rotreklová, V. Velčovský

Institute of Biophysics, Czechoslovak Academy of Sciences, Brno

Thyminedeoxyriboside (TdR) is generally accepted as a specific precursor of deoxyribonucleic acid (DNA). It may be incorporated into DNA either during DNA replication, i.e., in the course of the process leading to DNA reduplication, a fundamental prerequisite for the cell division; or during a process termed unscheduled DNA synthesis. DNA replication differs from unscheduled DNA synthesis in at least following three ways:

a) DNA replication occurs only in a limited period of interphase, in the *S*-phase. The unscheduled DNA synthesis seems to be independent of any phase of the cell cycle.
b) Many authors, e.g., Young and Hodas (1964), Schwartz et al. (1965), Yabro et al. (1965), Sinclair (1967) showed specific inhibition of DNA replication with hydroxyurea (HU), whilst according to Regan et al. (1968), Cleaver (1969), etc., the synthesis of unscheduled DNA remained unaffected in HU-treated cells. The cited findings suggest differences in the synthetic pathways of the two processes, in spite of the fact that the detailed mechanism of HU effect remains unknown (Young and Hodas 1964, Young et al. 1967).
c) The DNA replication is more or less inhibited by ionizing radiation, whereas the synthesis of unscheduled DNA may be induced by irradiation. The induction of unscheduled DNA synthesis with UV in HeLa cells was described as long as ten years ago by Rasmussen and Painter (1964), and two years later on also after X-irradiation (1966). Later on, this effect was observed by other authors, e.g., by Brent and Wheatley (1971), Roberts et al. (1971), Goodman and Potter (1972). The DNA synthesis induced with ionizing radiation was predominantly discussed in the terms of a repair of DNA radiation damage.

In intact cells, there are also some signs suggesting besides DNA replication another DNA turnover, occurring even in G_0 cells. In contrast to DNA replication, which takes hours, the mentioned DNA turnover proceeds throughout days. Pelc (1959) showed that DNA replication in regenerating rat liver was completed in about 8 hrs, whilst the DNA turnover in adult liver took more than 30 days. Pelc (1959) discussed the latter process as renewal of DNA molecules in G_0 cells.

The experiments described below would like to turn the attention to the rate of TdR utilization for DNA replication in cells under physiological conditions, in irradiated cells, and for the synthesis of unscheduled DNA in irradiated cells treated with HU.

---

* Cancer Research Institute, Academy of Sciences of German Democratic Republic, Berlin-Buch.

Material and Methods

The experiments were carried out on mice lymphosarcoma cells (LS/BL) in vitro. The cell suspension was prepared in HANKS'-solution (pH 7.4) and inactivated calf serum (2:1) containing 10^7 cells pro ml. The cells were labeled either with ^{3}H-TdR (24.2 Ci/mM, ÚVVVR Prag) or ^{14}C-TdR (43 mCi pro mM, Amersham). For the block of DNA replication 5 mM hydroxyurea was used. The cells were exposed to γ-rays of ^{60}Co. The incorporated radioisotope was detected either by means of β-spectrometer (Nuclear Chicago Mark 2) after treatment of the cells with NCS-solubilizer (Nuclear Chicago), or by autoradiography using standard stripping film procedure (Kodak AR. 10).

Results and Discussion

The rate of TdR utilization for DNA replication in cells under physiological conditions was tested when using 0.25, 0.5 and 2.0 μCi ^{14}C-TdR. The typical exponential incorporation curves were obtained, the linear parts of which are presented in Fig. 1. According

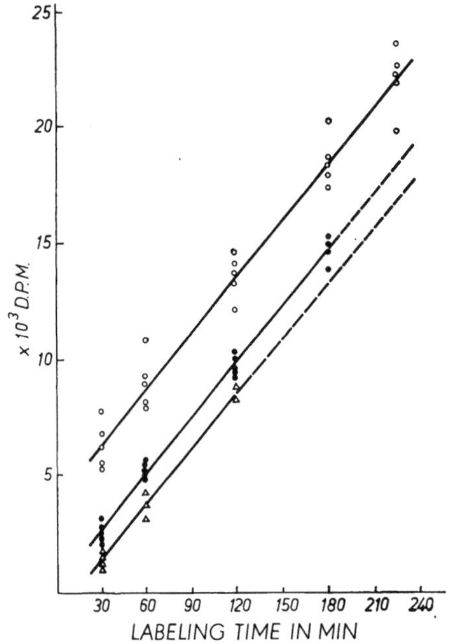

Fig. 1. Specific activity of DNA plotted against labeling time: △——△ — 0.25 μCi ^{14}C-TdR; •——• — 0.5 μCi ^{14}C-TdR; ○——○ — 2 μCi ^{14}C-TdR.

to these straight lines, the rate of TdR utilization for DNA replication was calculated. It was found that 1.2×10^{-17} mol of TdR were used for DNA replication in one minute. This value is in very good agreement with the data by CLEAVER and HOLFORD (1965), and by SALADINO and JOHNSON (1974).

The exposure of the cells to ionizing radiation produces a decrease in the uptake of TdR for DNA synthesis. In Fig. 2., a simplified imagination of the ^{3}H-TdR use for DNA replication is plotted against labeling time at different doses of γ-rays. In irradiated cells the rate of TdR utilization for DNA replication is lowered down with the dose:

from 1.2×10^{-17} mol TdR/min in nonirradiated cells to 0.5×10^{-17} mol TdR/min in the cells exposed to 5 krads (Tab. 1).
The ^{3}H-TdR incorporation into DNA of LS/BL lymphosarcoma cells treated with HU after the exposure to 5 krads was used for an attempt to estimate the amount of unscheduled DNA. Tritium activity in a cell was detected by means of autoradiography. When evaluating the autoradiographs, just the grains above a cell nucleus were counted and therefore the results allowed to consider nuclear DNA only.

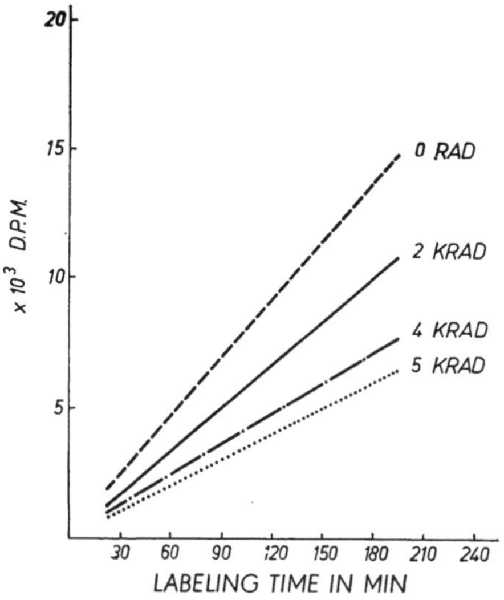

Fig. 2. Schematic imagination of the decrease of ^{3}H-TdR utilisation rate for DNA replication in nonirradiated cells (0 rad) and in the cells exposed to 2, 4 and 5 krads.

Table 1. Utilization rate of TdR.

Treatment	DNA Replication
Nonirradiated	1.2×10^{-17} mol TdR $\times$ min^{-1}
2 krads	0.89×10^{-17} mol TdR $\times$ min^{-1}
4 krads	0.64×10^{-17} mol TdR $\times$ min^{-1}
5 krads	0.54×10^{-17} mol TdR $\times$ min^{-1}
	Unscheduled DNA Synthesis
5 krads	2.48×10^{-18} mol TdR $\times$ min^{-1}

The histogram (Fig. 3) shows that in nonirradiated cells the HU-treatment did not block completely the ^{3}H-TdR incorporation into DNA. On average 8.4 grains per labeled cell were observed. The tritium activity bound in a cell during 2 hrs incubation, most probably the DNA residual replication in HU-treated nonirradiated cells, corresponded to the synthesis of about 0.5% of the total DNA. The irradiation of HU-treated cells stimulated ^{3}H-TdR incorporation into nuclear DNA by about tenfold (Fig. 4). The average graincount per labeled cell was 90.2. The difference between the average graincounts in irradiated and nonirradiated cells (81.8 grains) was used for the calcula-

tion of unscheduled DNA synthesis. According to this graincount it was calculated that during 2 hrs after irradiation there was synthesized a polynucleotide chain of the mass of 1.62×10^{11} daltons, of the length of 7.8×10^{8} Å, consisting of 2.3×10^{8} bases, out of which 5.9×10^{7} belonged to thymine.
The fundamental presupposition for this calculation consists in the presumption that the average base composition of the unscheduled DNA is approximately the same as that

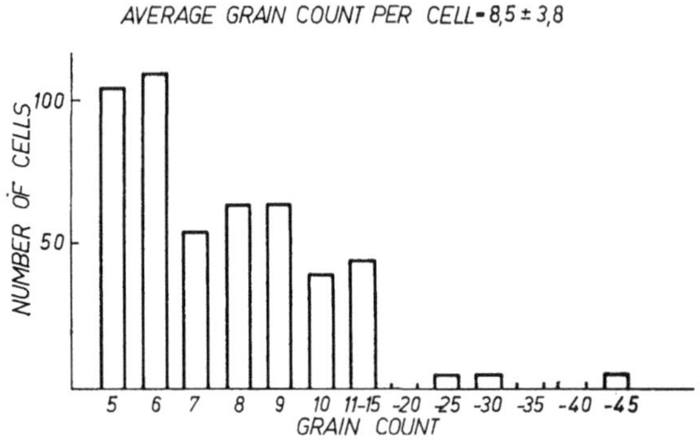

Fig. 3. Distribution of the ^{3}H-TdR labeled cells according to graincounts in the autoradiograph of nonirradiated cell population after HU-treatment.

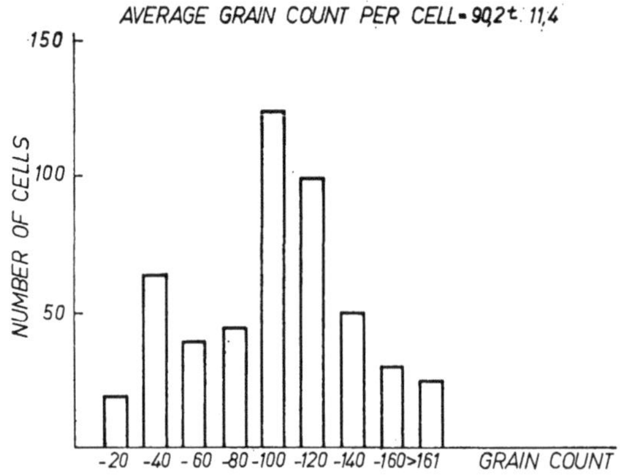

Fig. 4. Distribution of the ^{3}H-TdR labeled cells according to graincounts in the autoradiograph of irradiated cell population after HU-treatment.

of the replicative DNA. This presupposition may be a source of errors because the question of base sequences in unscheduled DNA remains still open. The rate of DNA replication decreases with the radiation dose (Fig. 2, Tab. 1). In spite of this fact, the DNA residual replication was in the calculation characterized with 8.4 grains, holding for nonirradiated cells and the probable radiation effect was neglected with the regard to the approximation used in the calculation.
The calculated 1.62×10^{11} daltons corresponds approximately to 5% of total DNA cell nucleus. Lukášová and Paleček (1972) found in the cells exposed to 6 krads about 5.8% of total DNA denatured by ionizing radiation. The amount of damaged DNA is

in good agreement with the amount of DNA the synthesis of which was induced by ionizing radiation.

The rate of TdR utilization in the process of unscheduled DNA synthesis in the cells exposed to 5 krads and treated with HU was about 2.48×10^{-18} mol TdR/min. This value is about five times smaller than that for DNA replication in nonirradiated and also smaller than those in irradiated cells (Tab. 1). The values of ^{3}H-TdR utilization rate in the processes of DNA replication and unscheduled DNA synthesis may be compared directly. The real synthetic rate of DNA replication and unscheduled DNA synthesis, however, depends on the number of points where the process takes place.

In LS/BL cells exposed to 5 krads about 32, 500 single-strand breaks (ssb) may be expected (personal communication Dr. Drášil, Institute of Biophysics, ČSAV, Brno). Assuming that the unscheduled DNA synthesis repairs the ssb, the real rate of unscheduled DNA synthesis at given ^{3}H-TdR utilization rate may differ in the extreme cases (ssb repaired simultaneously; ssb repaired consecutionally) approximately by the order of 10^4.

About a tenfold difference in the rate of TdR utilization between the synthesis of unscheduled DNA in irradiated cells and the above mentioned slow DNA turnover in G_0 cells renders a comparison of the two processes less probable.

Summary

The rate of TdR utilization for DNA replication was studied in the cells under physiological conditions, in irradiated cells (2, 4, and 5 krads), and for the synthesis of unscheduled DNA in irradiated cells (5 krads) treated with hydroxyurea (5 mM).

The rate of TdR utilization for DNA replication is reduced with the dose of γ-rays: from 1.2×10^{-17} mol TdR/min in nonirradiated cells to 0.5×10^{-17} mol TdR per min in cells exposed to 5 krads. The rate of TdR utilization in the process of unscheduled DNA synthesis was about 2.48×10^{-18} mol TdR/min.

References

[1] Brent, T. P., Wheatley, G. A.: Int. J. Rad. Biol. **19**, 339 (1971)
[2] Cleaver, J. E.: Rad. Res. **37**, 334 (1969)
[3] Cleaver, J. E., Holford, R. M.: Biochim. Biophys. Acta **103**, 654 (1965)
[4] Goodman, J. I., Potter, V. R.: Canc. Res. **32**, 767 (1972)
[5] Lukášová, E., Paleček, E.: Fol. biol. **18**, 307 (1972)
[6] Pelc, S. R.; Lab. Invest. **8**, 225 (1959)
[7] Rasmussen, R. E., Painter, R. B.: Nature **203**, 1360 (1964)
[8] Rasmussen, R. E., Painter, R. B.: J. Cell Biol. **29**, 11 (1966)
[9] Regan, J. P., Trosko, J. E., Carrier, W. L.: Biophys. J. **8**, 319 (1968)
[10] Roberts, J. J., Pascoe, J. M., Smith, B. A., and Crathorn, A. N.: Chem. Biol. Interct. **3**, 49 (1971)
[11] Saladino, C. F., Johnson, H. A.: Exp. Cell Res. **85**, 248 (1974)
[12] Schwartz, H. S., Garofalo, M., Sternberg, S. S., and Philips, F. S.: Cancer Res. **25**, 1867 (1965)
[13] Sinclair, W. K.,: Cancer Res. **27**, 297 (1967)
[14] Yabro, J. W., Kennedy, B. J., and Barnum, C. P.: Proc. Natl. Acad. Sci. US **53**, 1033 (1965)
[15] Young, C. W., and Hodas, S.: Science **146**, 1172 (1964)
[16] Young, C. W., Schochetman, G., and Karnofsky, D. A.: Cancer Res. **27**, 526 (1967)

Comparative Evaluation of the DNA Repair Contribution to the Recovery of the Viability of Bacteria and the Eukaryotic Cells after Irradiation

V. D. Zhestyanikov

Laboratory of Radiation Cytology, Institute of Cytology, Academy of Sciences of the USSR, Leningrad, USSR

A large body of evidence obtained on bacteria demonstrated a close correlation between repair processes at the cellular and molecular levels. It should be taken for granted that the DNA repair is an important factor in the recovery of cell viability of microorganisms (for review see: Zhestyanikov, 1968, 1970; Smith, 1971; Town, Smith and Kaplan, 1973). Most significant evidence was derived from experiments on mutants of microorganisms in which the survival and DNA repair using physico-chemical methods were investigated in parallel.

Results obtained during a few recent years, findings of our laboratory among thems, support the conclusion that DNA repair plays the essential role in recovery of the cell viability after irradiation and action of chemical mutagens and carcinogens.

DNA repair and survival of bacteria

At present about 25 mutations in *Escherichia coli* are known to affect the DNA repair (see Table 1). Mutations in all these genes result in the increase of cell radiosensitivity. Similar data were obtained in experiments with other bacteria and eukariotic microorganisms. Mutations responsible for the increased radiosensitivity and inability to repair

Table 1. List of genes affecting DNA repair and radiosensitivy in *Escherichia coli**.

Genes	Approximate map location	Controlled function	Sensitivity	
			to UV-light	to X-rays
uvr A	91	ER: incision; regulatory	+	−
uvr B	17	function	+	−
uvr C	42	Control of ligase activity after incision (prevention of joining 3'OH−5'PO_4); incision	+	−
uvr D	84	ER: possibly, repair synthesis; PR	+	±
uvr E	84	ER: repair synthesis; regulatory function (?)	+	±
pol A1 (pol A107, *res* 1)	85	Structural gene for DNA polymerase I. ER: repair synthesis by short patches (10−30 nucleotides); PR: possibly, de novo synthesis; fast repair of DNA SSB	+	+

Table 1. (continued)

Genes	Approximate map location	Controlled function	Sensitivity	
			to UV-light	to X-rays
pol B	2	Structural gene for DNA polymerase II. ER: repair synthesis in the absence of DNA polymerases I and III; PR	—	—
pol C (*dna* E)	4	Structural gene for DNA polymerase III. ER: repair synthesis by long patches (1000 nucleotides); PR: de novo synthesis (?)	+	+
lig	51	Structural gene for DNA ligase; ER; PR; SSB DNA Repair	+	+
lex A	90	ER; PR: "SOS"-repair, de novo synthesis; slow repair of DNA SSB; regulation of cell division	+	+ some strains: —
exr B	90	Regulation of cell division	+	?
zab (*lex* B, *tif*)	58	PR: "SOS"-repair	+	?
xth A	38	Structural gene for endonuclease II and exonuclease III	+	±
lon	10	Cell division	+	+
ras	9	?	+	±
ror A	60	?	—	+
rer	84	Replication of damaged DNA in the presence of repairable damage	+	+
rec A	58	Complete recombinational deficiency. ER: repair synthesis by long patches; PR: recombination and "SOS"-repair; slow repair of DNA SSB	+	+
rec B *rec* C	60 60	Structural genes for ATP-dependent endo- exo- nuclease. ER; PR: recombination; slow repair of DNA SSB	+ +	+ +
rec F (*uvr* F)	82	PR: recombination	+	±

* Clark, 1973; Town, Smith and Kaplan, 1973; Clark and Canesan, 1975; Bachmann, Low and Taylor, 1976; Tomilin, 1977.

+, ±, — increased sensitivity, moderate sensitivity, resistance to radiation (respectively);

ER — excision repair of UV-induced pyrimidine dimers; PR — post-replication repair; SSB — single-strand breaks.

the DNA structural and information integrity were described for *Salmonella typhimurium* (SKAVRONSKAYA, 1974), *Haemophilus influenzae* (SMALL, 1975), *Bacillus subtilis* (MAZZA et al., 1975). More than 30 radiosensitivity mutations are known in the yeast *Saccharomyces cerevisiae* (HAYNES, 1975; ZAKHAROV, 1976).

Only part of genes controlling the DNA repair processes in *E. coli* code enzymes. The majority of the genes code the synthesis of products the function of which is not yet clearly defined. It appears that many of them perform the function of regulatory proteins.

Some enzymes and gene products, along with the DNA repair processes control replication and recombination in intact cells. So *pol* C (*dna* E) gene, structural gene for the replication enzyme DNA polymerase III, plays the important role in the DNA repair after irradiation. In our laboratory N. V. TOMILIN found out that DNA polymerase III is involved in the recovery of viability of γ-ray-irradiated *E. coli* (TOMILIN, 1974). Later on it was shown by the alkaline sucrose gradient technique that at permissive temperature (active DNA polymerase III) the strain *E. coli* BT 1026 *dna* E^{ts} *pol* A1 repairs effectively single-strand breaks of DNA while at non-permissive temperature (*dna* E^{-}-phenotype) these lesions are not repaired (ZHESTYANIKOV et al., 1975). Moreover, DNA polymerase III participates both in excision repair of UV-light-induced dimers performing the repair synthesis by long patches (YOUNGS a. SMITH, 1973) and in combination with DNA polymerase I in post-replication gap-filling in UV-irradiated cells (TOMILIN and SVETLOVA, 1974; SEDGWICK and BRIDGES, 1974; TAIT, HARRIS and SMITH, 1974).

In 1971 W. FANGMAN and M. RUSSEL found that active product of *dna* B gene controlling the elongation of DNA during replication is involved in recovery of the *E. coli* viability after the action of X-ray-irradiation.

Recently we investigated the role of *dna* G gene controlling initiation of the OKAZAKI-pieces synthesis in the repair of γ-ray-induced lesions in *E. coli*. Some of results are presented in Fig. 1 illustrating the survival of *E. coli* PC3, sedimentation profiles and elimination of DNA single-strand breaks after irradiation. Survival of the strain carrying *dna* G thermosensitive mutation depends on temperature conditions. The survival was higher when bacteria were kept at a permissive temperature of 30 °C. Preliminary maintenance of irradiated cells at 43 °C for 2—4 hours and subsequent incubation at 30 °C leads to the decrease of their survival. The DNA degradation and synthesis correlate with the survival (ZHESTYANIKOV and SAVEL'EVA, 1976). As seen from Fig 1b, the molecular weight of single-strand DNA which reduced after irradiation is restored in condition of *dna* G^{+}-phenotype under post radiation growth at 30 °C and is not restored at 43 °C. In our experiments γ-ray-irradiation at a dose of 15 krad induced 7 breaks in PC3 double-strand genome. These breaks are completely eliminated at 30 °C (Fig. 1c).

In our laboratory we studied the question whether other genes controlling the DNA replication take part in the repair of γ-ray-induced DNA single-strand breaks and in the post-replication gap-filling in UV-irradiated cells. The results are summarized in Table 2. Besides the above evidence one can see that the thermosensitive mutation in *dna* G gene at non-permissive temperature prevents from post-replication repair. Mutations in *dna* A (in LC 179 strain) and *dna* B (in CR 34 strain) do not affect the rejoining of DNA single-strand breaks and post-replication gap-filling.

It must be added that in instances when a study was made of the DNA repair and survival a complete correlation was observed between them.

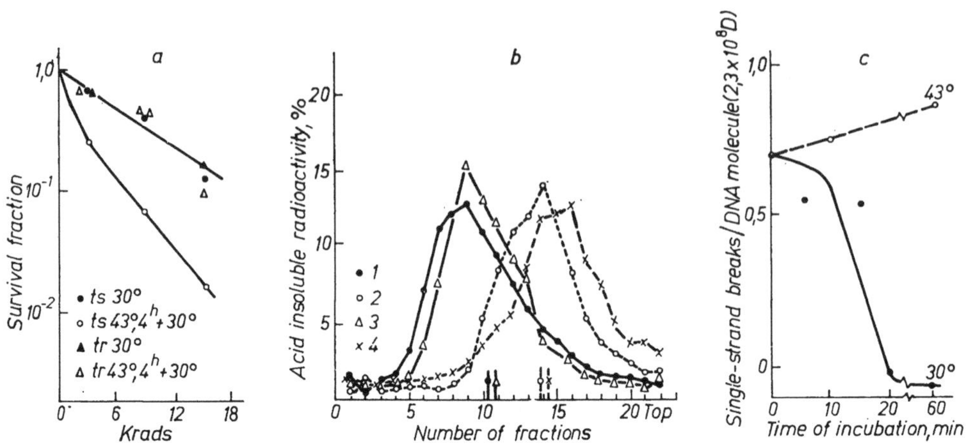

Fig. 1. Survival (a) and repair of DNA single-strand breaks (b, c) in *E. coli* PC3 *dna* G^{ts} after γ-ray-irradiation.

a. Strains PC3 *dna* G^{ts} and its tr-revertant after irradiation were placed on nutrient agar medium at 30° or preliminary for 4 h at 43 °C. All the remaining time they were kept at 30 °C until the formation of macrocolonies.

b. Sedimentation profiles and weight-average molecular weights (vertical lines) of DNA from *E. coli* PC3 *dna* G^{ts}. 1 — Unirradiated control, 2 — 14.5 krad with no incubation, 3.4 —14.5 krad, reincubation for 60 min at 30 ° and 43 °C respectively.

c. Number of DNA single-strand breaks in PC3 *dna* G^{ts} strain during postradiation incubation at 30° and 43°.

For details see ZHESTYANIKOV and SAVEL'EVA 1976.

Table 2. Repair of DNA radiation damage with participation of gene products controlling DNA replication in *Escherichia coli.*

E. *coli* K 12 strain	Thermosensitive mutation *dna*	Failure in repair of γ-ray-induced DNA single-strand breaks* at non-permissive temperature	Failure in repair of post-replication gaps* in UV-irradiated cells at non-permissive temperature
LC 179	A	—	—
CR 34	B	—	—
E 279	B	not investigated	+**
BT 1026	E	+***	+****
PC 3	G	+***	+***
JW 187	G	+	not investigated

* Restoration of DNA molecular weight determined by alkaline sucrose gradients sedimentation technique was used as a criterion of repair of DNA single-strand breaks and post-replication gaps (for details see SVETLOVA et al., 1974).

** JOHNSON, 1975.

*** ZHESTYANIKOV et al., 1975.

**** TOMILIN and SVETLOVA, 1974.

The rule of causal relationship between the radioresistance and DNA repair in bacteria almost has no exclusion. This is supported not only by the above data also by examples which on the surface lack such relationship.
It is found that thymine and amino acid starvation in auxotrophic *E. coli* uvr^+ decreases the ability to excise cyclobutane pyrimidine dimers from DNA. However the UV-resistance of the bacteria was not reduced. On the contrary, it enhanced in the *E. coli* uvr^- strain that had undergone amino acid or thymine prestarvation before irradiation. Changes of these properties (repair of DNA and radioresistance) was determined by compensatory development of the capacity to fill post-replication gaps in the daughter DNA (SEDLIAKOVÁ et al., 1973).
In wild cells of *Micrococcus luteus* excision repair of UV-induced dimers and post-replication repair of DNA were most efficient (Table 3). In a UV-sensitive mutant

Table 3. UV-resistance and DNA repair in *Micrococcus luteus* cells*.

M. luteus strain	Resistance to UV-light	Excision repair of pyrimidine dimers	Repair of post-replication gaps
ATCC 4698 (wild type)	+	+	+++
G7	—	—	+
Trf (G7)	+	—	++

* For details see ZHEREBTSOV and TOMILIN, 1975.

M. luteus G7 the first mechanisms is missing and the second is weakly pronounced. The Trf (G7) transformant just like parental UV-sensitive mutant is not capable to excise dimers from DNA. However it shows the same UV-resistance as the wild type. The latter is due to the efficient post-replication repair of DNA (Table 3; Fig. 2) (ZHEREBTSOV and TOMILIN, 1975).

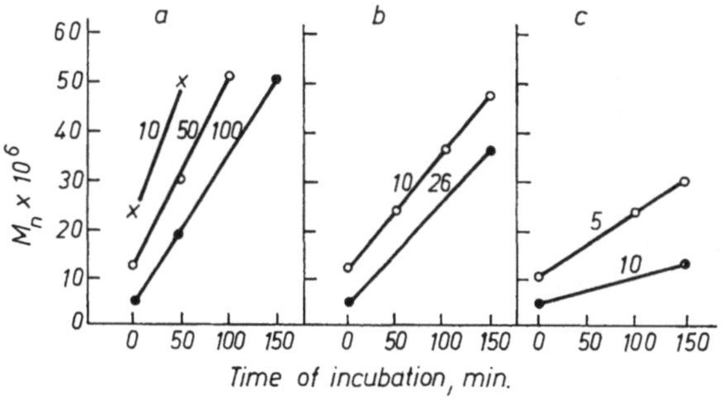

Fig. 2. Increase of the number-average molecular weight of post-replication DNA fragments depending on the time of incubation of *Micrococcus luteus* irradiated with UV-light.
a. *M. luteus* ATCC 4698, wild type; b. *M. luteus* Trf (G7); c. *M. luteus* G7.
UV-light doses indicate near each line (from ZHEREBTSOV and TOMILIN, 1975. Biochim. et biophys. Acta, **383**, 16—22).

Thus the level of bacterial cells resistance to irradiation is defined by the common contribution of activities of all cell repair systems.

If this is true most rare case of incomplete correlation between repair processes at the molecular and cellular levels can be accounted for by existence of a few DNA repair mechanisms, in addition to the excision repair and post-replication repair each having several pathways and branches.

Let us consider from this viewpoint the peculiarities of repair processes in *E. coli* mutants B_{S-1} and $B_{S-1}\gamma$ R. The latter mutant was isolated in conditions of continuous γ-ray-irradiation of B_{S-1} (ZHESTYANIKOV, 1966). In some of its properties mutant $B_{S-1}\gamma$ R *lex* A is similar to the parental strain B_{S-1} *lex* A (it is sensitive to UV-light, nitrogen mustard, mitomycine C, does not reactivate UV-irradiated phage T1, does not excise pyrimidine dimers from DNA) while in other it shows a phenotypical resemblance to the radioresistant strain *E. coli* B/r (it is resistant to γ-ray-irradiation, methyl methanesulfonate and hydroxylamine). Mutant $B_{S-1}\gamma$ R is three-five times more resistant to UV-light than B_{S-1}. This circumstance seems to be due to a more efficient post-replication repair of DNA (Table 4). Strain $B_{S-1}\gamma$ R was found to fill 90% of post-replication gaps resulting from UV-irradiation with the doses 2—6 $J \cdot m^{-2}$, while mutant B_{S-1} repaired only 60% of the gaps (SVETLOVA, TOMILIN and ZHESTYANIKOV, 1974).

Table 4. DNA repair in *Escherichia coli* B strains.

Radiation dose	Incubation time, min	Fraction of repaired single-strand breaks (I) and post-replication gaps (II), %%*		
		B_{S-1}	$B_{S-1}\gamma$ R	B/r
I 15 krad	45	no repair	100	100
30 krad	60—80	no repair	30	95
II 2 $J \cdot m^{-2}$	70	59	91	not
6 $J \cdot m^{-2}$	70	65	89	investigated

* See footnote to Table 2.

By its repairability γ-ray-induced DNA single-strand breaks *E. coli* $B_{S-1}\gamma$ R differs from as much radioresistant strain B/r. Mutant $B_{S-1}\gamma$ R repaired breaks completely only after irradiation with 15 krad whereas two-fold increase of the dose reduced the repair capacity (Table 4) (SVETLOVA et al., 1974). The same results were obtained from study of another *lex* A mutant of *E. coli* (SEDGWICK and BRIDGES, 1972).

Some peculiar traits of *lex* A mutants suggest the existence of a DNA repair mechanism due to which irradiated cells survive irrespective of non-repaired single-strand breaks.

DNA repair in model systems

Reliable evidence for the existence of a particular biochemical mechanism can be provided only if it reconstructed in a non-cellular model system. The DNA repair was able reproduced in semi- in vitro system in toluene-treated cells. Even first such experiments showed that UV-endonuclease, DNA polymerase I and DNA ligase are indispensable for the excision repair of UV-light-irradiation transforming DNA (HEIJNEKER et al., 1971), and the two last enzymes for the repair of X-ray-irradiated DNA (LAIPIS and GANESAN, 1972).

Initiation of the excision repair in a UV-irradiated cells depends on the activity of the *uvr* A and *uvr* B genes since these mutations block the repair process as a whole.

In case UV-irradiated infections DNA of phage λ is introduced into *E. coli* uvr^- its survival (plaque-forming ability) in these cells is much lower than in uvr^+ strain. In vitro treatment of λ-DNA with UV-endonuclease from *M. luteus* enhanced the ability to form negative colonies up to survival level in uvr^+ cells (Table 5) (TOMILIN and MOSEVITSKAYA, 1974, 1975).

Table 5. Recovery of infectivity of λ-DNA treated with UV-endonuclease from.
Micrococcus luteus and measured in *Escherichia coli* K12 Ca^{++}-treated cells.
(TOMILIN and MOSEVITSKAYA, 1975).

E. coli strain	D_{37} ($J \cdot m^{-2}$)	
	Without enzyme	With enzyme
AB 1157 uvr^+	27	20
AB 1886 *uvr* A	5.5	18
AB 1885 *uvr* B	6.5	18
AB 1884 *uvr* C	9	20

Complete reconstruction of the repair of UV-irradiated DNA was performed in vitro by N. V. TOMILIN. In non-cellular system, containing UV-endonuclease and DNA polymerase I from *M. luteus* and ATP-dependent DNA ligase of phage T4, cyclobutane dimers of pyrimidines were fully removed and the molecular weight of linear molecules of λ-DNA was restored (Fig. 3a). Restitution of the DNA physical integrity (without controlling the biological activity) succesively treated with the above three enzymes was reconstructed also on a model of plasmid ColE1 DNA. In this instance complete repair of incision breaks was observed up to the UV-dose of 120 $J \cdot m^{-2}$ (TOMILIN, 1976). Similar results were obtained with RF ⌀X 174-DNA (HEIJNEKER, 1975) and transforming DNA of *B. subtilis* (HAMILTON et al., 1975).

The experimental evidence demonstrating the reconstruction of DNA repair in vitro is of interest from another point of view. It was obvious that for a complete recovery of some biological properties of UV-damaged DNA molecules only three enzyme activities are needed, which, however, should be used not simultaneously but in succession (this provide for a recovery of the transforming DNA biological activity in vitro (HEIJNEKER et al., 1971)]. This fact as well as ~10 enzymes and non-identified gene products required for DNA complete repair in a cell irradiated with UV-light indicate that the bulk of these gene products perform regulatory functions and coordinate the work of most essential repair enzymes in time and space (TOMILIN, 1977).

UV-endonuclease exhibits a non-specificity when recognizing besides cyclobutane pyrimidine dimers, apurinic sites in the DNA (TOMILIN, 1974). In the supercoiled DNA of phage λ with depurinations induced with heat and acid UV-endonuclease from *M. luteus* resulted in the formation of nicks transferring the supercoiled λ-DNA into the open form. In neutral sucrose the latter sediments at a lower rate than the first one. The addition to a reactive mixture containing depurinated λ-DNA and UV-endonuclease of heterologous DNA irradiated with UV-light reduced the formation of λ-DNA open molecules (experiments of N. V. Tomilin, T. V. Mosevitskaya and E. B. Pavel-tschuk). Thus competition for UV-endonuclease between UV-irradiated and depurinated DNA indicates that the incision enzyme — UV-endonuclease — participates in the repair of depurinated DNA.

At the same time, the effect of UV-endonuclease from *M. luteus* on depurinated DNA does not cause a recovery of its biological activity (ability to form negative colonies) of infectious λ-DNA but even increases its further inactivation (data of N. V. Tomilin and T. V. Mosevitskaya). This indicates a more complex repair of depurinated DNA in the cell as compared to the DNA irradiated with UV-light.

The physical integrity of depurinated DNA is recovered in vitro in the system identical

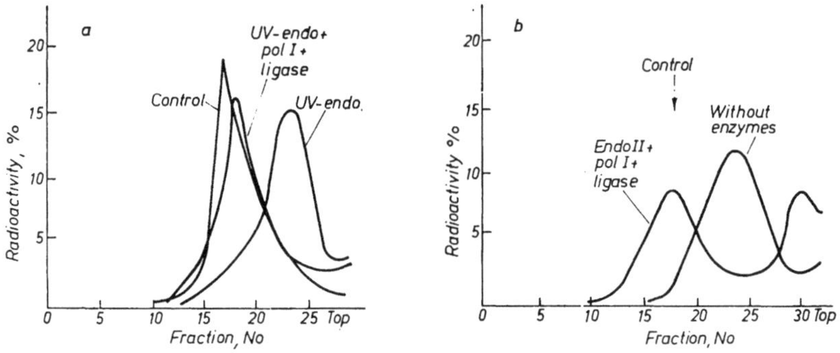

Fig. 3. In vitro restoration of molecul weight of linear molecules of λ-DNA (reconstruction) after UV-irradiation with 60 J · m^{-2} (a) and depurination (1.5 apurinic sites per one λ-DNA) (b).

a. 1. Production of UV-irradiated λ-DNA: the mixture consisting of 0.05 ml ^{3}H-λ-DNA ($5 \cdot 10^4$ cpm, 5 μg) in 0.2 ml of 0.4 M Tris-HCl buffer, pH 7.7 was irradiated with UV-light (60 J · m^{-2}).

2. Treatment with UV-endonuclease: the incubation mixture consisting of UV-irradiated λ-DNA, 0.05 ml UV-endonuclease from *Micrococcus luteus* (F IV) and 0.05 ml distilled water was incubated at 37° for 60 min.

3. Reconstruction: the mixture consisting of 0.05 ml UV-irradiated λ-DNA, 0.05 ml UV-endonuclease (F IV, ~ 0,08 units), 0.05 ml DNA polymerase I from *M. luteus* (F IV, ~ 4 units), 0.05 ml DNA ligase of T4 phage (F V, ~ 1.5 units), 0.05 ml of mixture containing Mg^{++} (final concentration in incubation mixture — 10 mM), ATP (final concentration 0.5 mM) and four deoxynucleotidetriphosphate (final concentration of each 30 mM) was incubated at 37 °C for 60 min.

b. 1. Production of depurinated DNA: the mixture consisting of 0.15 ml ^{14}C-λ-DNA ($15 \cdot 10^4$ cpm, 15 μg), 0.15 ml of 0.01 M citrate buffer with 0.1 M NaCl, pH 5.0 and 0.2 ml of 0.4 M Tris-HCl buffer pH 5.9 was heated at 70 °C for 24 min.

2. Reconstruction: composition of incubation mixture — 0.05 ml of depurinated DNA, 0.05 ml of endonuclease II (F III, ~ 40 units) for the remaing components and manipulations see a. 3.

0.1 ml of each sample was layered on to surface of a linear 5—20% alkaline sucrose gradient (4.8 ml). Ultracentrifugation was performed in a rotor SW65 of Spinko L2-65 centrifuge: 50000 rpm for 60 min (a) or 80 min (b) at 20 °C (N. V. Tomilin's-data).

to that restored in the case of UV-irradiated DNA, with UV-endonuclease from *M. luteus* as the recognizing enzyme (N. V. TOMILIN's-data). Moreover, restoration of the molecular weight of depurinated DNA involves of another endonuclease from *M. luteus* — endonuclease II as a recognizing enzyme. This enzyme isolated by N. V. TOMILIN and L. S. BARENFELD, just like endonuclease II from *E. coli* (HADI and GOLDTHWAIT, 1971), has a molecular weight of 30000 daltons and causes breaks in DNA containing apurinic sites and bases modified by γ-ray-irradiation. In the in vitro system endonuclease II in combination with DNA polymerase I and DNA ligase repairs depurinated DNA (Fig. 3b). In the same system N. V. TOMILIN reconstructed the repair of DNA containing bases modified by ionizing radiation.

Consequently, the experiments on model systems indicate convincingly that the DNA repair is essential for the recovery of biological properties of an irradiated cell. Needless to say not all details of this elaborate cellular process are elucidated which is evident from the experiment on recovery of the viability of infectious depurinated λ-DNA. However the achievements in this field are abvious.

DNA repair and recovery of viability of higher eukaryotic cells

It appears that the dependence between the DNA repair and the recovery of viability of irradiation-damaged cell is on a whole rather regular. Evidence given below show conclusively that these regularities hold both for prokaryotic cells and for the cells of higher eukaryotic organism. In the latter case however the solution of the problem is not unambiguous. A number of discrepancies are known to exist between data obtained at the molecular and cellular levels from experiments on mammalian and plant cells. It is likely that there occur difficulties of two kinds. The first is that higher eukaryots, unlike microorganisms, are known to have a small number of mutations involving DNA repair and radiosensitivity. In human these mutations induce hereditary diseases such as Xeroderma pigmentosum, FANCONI's-anemia, ataxia telangiectasia and possibly BLOOM's syndrome (for reviews see GERMAN, 1972; CLEAVER, 1974; ZAKHAROV, 1976; PATERSON and SMITH, 1976). In plant cells mutations of radiosensitivity are not yet found. The second difficulty is partly connected with the first and partly is explained by the fact that until now it is unknown whether animal and plant cells possess only those repair mechanisms that operate in microorganisms or they are provided with some especial mechanisms. The latter is not excluded if we take into account a more complex organization of genetic material in cells of higher eukaryotes. Hence unequivocal of evaluations of the role of given lethal lesions effects of irradiation. Equally, it is still impossible to assess the contribution of separate repair mechanisms to radiosensitivity of the cell. Meanwhile both these circumstance are especially essential for mammalian cells. In relation with the above is the problem of radiosensitivy control (control of DNA repair). This is important, among other things, for the effectiveness of malignant tumor radiotherapy and for the treatment of the aforementioned hereditary diseases considered to be precancerous.

A small number of mutations known in man stimulated studies on the effect of DNA repair inhibitors and involved cell processes. One of such agents — caffeine — that exerted an inhibitory effect on repair processes in bacteria (for review see ZHESTYANIKOV, 1970). It was suggested that by blocking the recovery caffeine type substances would mimic mutations in genes controlling the DNA repair. This assumption however was corraborated but partially which is due to a most intricate action of caffeine in irradiated plant and mammalian cells.

A great number of investigations carried out by different authors contain contradictory evidence. Moreover there occur lots of discrepancies in results obtained in the same laboratory and even on the same test subject.

In our laboratory the caffeine effects were studied experimentally on plant and human cells (Zhestyanikov, 1975).

In X-ray-irradiated diploid and tetraploid buckwheat roots cells and *Vicia faba* roots caffeine increases the frequency of chromosome aberrations (Krupnova and Seitkhodzhaev, 1974; Krupnova and Alekhina, 1974). This effect is accounted for by the inhibition of cell recovery process. In γ-ray-irradiated meristematic root culture of *V. faba* cells caffeine is found to inhibit stimulated incorporation of labelled thymidine at a non synthesized stage of the cell cycle (unscheduled synthesis of DNA). Similar effects are observed under the treatment with nitrogen mustard, activated carcinogene 7-bromomethyl-benz[a]anthracene and N-methyl-N'-nitro-N-nitrosoguanidine (Fig. 4) (G. F. Krupnova's-data).

In human lymphocytes caffeine increased the frequency of X-ray-induced chromosome aberrations at S-G_2 stage but not at the G_0-G_1 stage (Haikazyan, Mikhelson and Zhestyanikov, 1974). In non-stimulated leucocytes caffeine inhibits unscheduled synthesis of DNA after irradiation with UV-light (Genter, Noskova and Mikhelson, 1974) and in γ-ray-irradiated PHA-stimulated cells at the G_2 stage it inhibits the repair of DNA single-strand breaks (Haikazyan, Mikhelson and Zhestyanikov, 1973).

It can be concluded that in the experiments on human lymphocytes complete correlation was found between the results obtained at the molecular and cellular levels. These data are at variance with the findings for HeLa cells.

In HeLa Zh-63 cells caffeine decreases the survival and unscheduled synthesis of DNA after UV-light and ionizing radiation (Zhestyanikov, Semenova and Volkova, 1974; Semenova, Volkova and Zhestyanikov, 1974). But this agent affects the repair of DNA single-strand breaks induced by γ-ray-irradiation in different ways depending on the radiation dose. At irradiation of HeLa Zh-63 cells with light doses (1 krad) caffeine inhibits distinctly the rejoining of single-strand breaks (Pinto et al., 1974) while at irradiation with heavy doses (20 krad) repair in the presence of caffeine is efficient (Vikhanskaya and Pinto, 1976), similar data were received by other investigators (Lehmann, 1972a; Kleijer et al., 1973). Caffeine does not inhibit the repair of DNA double-strand breaks (Vikhanskaya and Pinto, 1976).

Up to now two contradictory facts in experiments demonstrating the action of caffeine on the repair of DNA breaks are not elucidated. Therefore it is not clear what repair mechanism inhibition causes the caffeine-induced increase in the frequency of chromosome aberrations and diminishing of the survival of irradiated cells.

It is not inconceivable that the effect of this agent is convected with its influence on some other processes. Its effect on post-replication repair after γ-ray-irradiation was specially investigated.

The phenomenology of the post-replication repair in UV-irradiated mammalian cells is the same as that in bacteria. However in mammalian cells gap-filling is accomplished via de novo synthesis but not by recombination exchanges between sister duplexes (Lehmann, 1972b). Besides the repair is possible due to a bypass of lesions without gaps in nascent DNA which occurs as a rule long time after irradiation (Lehmann and

Kirk-Bell, 1972; Buhl et al., 1973) or in the course of replication (Higgins, Kato and Strauss, 1976). It is shown that the repair of UV-induced post-replication gaps is inhibited with caffeine (for review see Lehmann, 1974).

Post-replication repair after X-ray-irradiation was detected in Chinese hamster cells (Körner and Malz, 1973, 1975; Körner, Malz and Günter, 1974). Cells irradiated and then incubated for 60 min to repair DNA single-strand breaks were labeled with ^{3}H-thymidine. The analysis of newly synthesized DNA indicates that it has a smaller single-strand molecular weight than that from unirradiated cells. During subsequent incubation in the growth medium the molecular weight of pulse-labeled material approaches that of the unirradiated control. The similarity between the discovered phenomenon and the process of gap-filling in UV-irradiated cells permits the suggestion

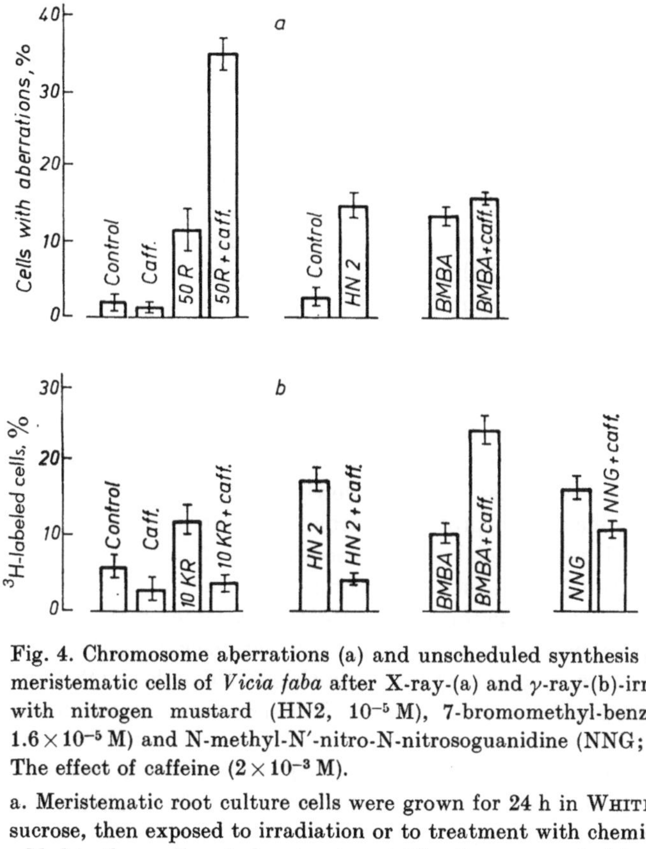

Fig. 4. Chromosome aberrations (a) and unscheduled synthesis of DNA (b) in cultured meristematic cells of *Vicia faba* after X-ray-(a) and γ-ray-(b)-irradiation and treatment with nitrogen mustard (HN2, 10^{-5} M), 7-bromomethyl-benz[a]anthracene (BMBA, 1.6×10^{-5} M) and N-methyl-N'-nitro-N-nitrosoguanidine (NNG; 5×10^{-3} M).
The effect of caffeine (2×10^{-3} M).

a. Meristematic root culture cells were grown for 24 h in White's-medium devoided of sucrose, then exposed to irradiation or to treatment with chemical agents. Caffeine was added to the medium before treatment. Fixation was made 2 h after treatment. Bridges and fragments in the first mitosis after treatment were taken into account. 1500 cells were counted up for each variant.

b. Cut off roots were grown for 24 h in White's-medium devoided of sucrose. Hydroxyurea (2×10^{-3} M) and caffeine were added together to the medium 2 h before treatment. ^{3}H-thymidine (5 μCi/ml) was added for 1 h after treatment. Emulsion of "P" type was exposed for 8 weeks at 4 °C. Cells containing 8–30 grains above the nucleus (unscheduled synthesis of DNA) were taken into account, 1500 cells were counted up for each variant (G. F. Krupnova's-data).

that in X-ray-irradiated cells newly synthesized DNA contains gaps. As in the case of UV-irradiation these gaps are filled via de novo synthesis.

In our laboratory R. I. Pinto and F. L. Vikhanskaya repeated experiments on HeLa Zh-63 cells according to the protocol described. After γ-ray-irradiation with the doses 1—5 krad, however, newly synthesized DNA had the same molecular weight as DNA in unirradiated cells. The result was the same when pulse-labeling with ^{3}H-thymidine was performed immediately after irradiation or, as in the experiments of I. Körner and W. Malz with Chinese hamster cells, after a 60-min incubation in non-radioactive medium. Consequently in HeLa Zh-63 cells on a parental strains containing γ-ray-induced lesions DNA was synthesized without gaps. Identical data were obtained in experiments with X-ray-irradiated HeLa 63 cells (I. Körner a. W. Malz, personal communication). In the other words, in γ-ray-irradiated HeLa cells, unlike the cell of Chinese hamster, no substrate for post-replication repair was found.

These results may be interpreted in two ways. Either in γ-ray-irradiated HeLa cells act mechanisms of damage bypass [similar to that described in experiments of A. R. Lehmann and S. Kirk-Bell (1972) and S. N. Buhl, R. B. Setlow and J. D. Regan (1973) or in experiments of N. Higgins, K. Kato and B. Strauss (1976)] or the post-replication gap-filling occurs during pulse labeling which lasts 45 min in conditions of experiments with HeLa Zh-63 cells.

The second assumption could be checked in experiments in which caffeine was added to medium simultaneously with ^{3}H-thymidine. Since caffeine inhibits post-replication repair the molecular weight of nascent DNA was expected to decrease on comparison with DNA synthesized during labeling without caffeine.

In these experiments in addition to the effect of γ-ray-irradiation, the action of UV-light, 7-bromomethyl-benz[a]anthracene and 2-aminofluorene was investigated. The results of the experiments are presented in Fig. 5.

The presence of caffeine in UV-irradiated cells during labeling with ^{3}H-thymidine results in a decrease of the molecular weight of newly synthesized DNA. This is evidenced by shifts of the sedimentation profile towards light fractions as compared to the sedimentation profile of DNA pulse labeled in the absence of caffeine (as shown earlier in UV-irradiated HeLa Zh-63 cells post-replication repair proceeded in the same manner as in experiments of other investigators). The effect of caffeine on the magnitute of a newly synthesized DNA molecule in unirradiated cell was specially tested. Since it was found that caffeine inhibits insignificantly the synthesis of daughter DNA in sedimentogrames sedimentation profiles of DNA from caffeine-treated non-irradiated cells were presented as a control.

The results of experiments with UV-irradiated cells (Fig. 5a) are in accordance with the assumption and indicate that part of the gaps are filled and that caffeine inhibits this process during 45-min pulse-labeling.

Similar data were obtained from experiments on cells treated with 7-bromomethyl-benz[a]anthracene (Fig. 5b).

However after γ-ray-irradiation and the action of 2-aminofluorene (Fig. 5c and 5d) the presence of caffeine during pulse-labeling does not lead to shift in sedimentation profiles as compared to profiles typical of DNA synthesized in the absence of caffeine.

Thus in experiments with HeLa cells no post-replication gaps were found to form as a result of γ-ray-irradiation. From this it is inferred that the effect of caffeine on the survival and formation of chromosome aberrations in X-ray-irradiated cells cannot be

explained by its effect on the DNA post-replication repair. It is not excluded that caffeine affects some still unknown repair processes. It might be an excision repair of bases modified by ionizing radiation. A wrong repair of DNA single-strand breaks or double-strand breaks is likely to proceed in the presence of caffeine. Such error repair may lead to chromosome aberrations and increase in the lethality of irradiated cells.
The results of our investigation of caffeine effects in experiments on plant and human cells are summarized in Table 6.

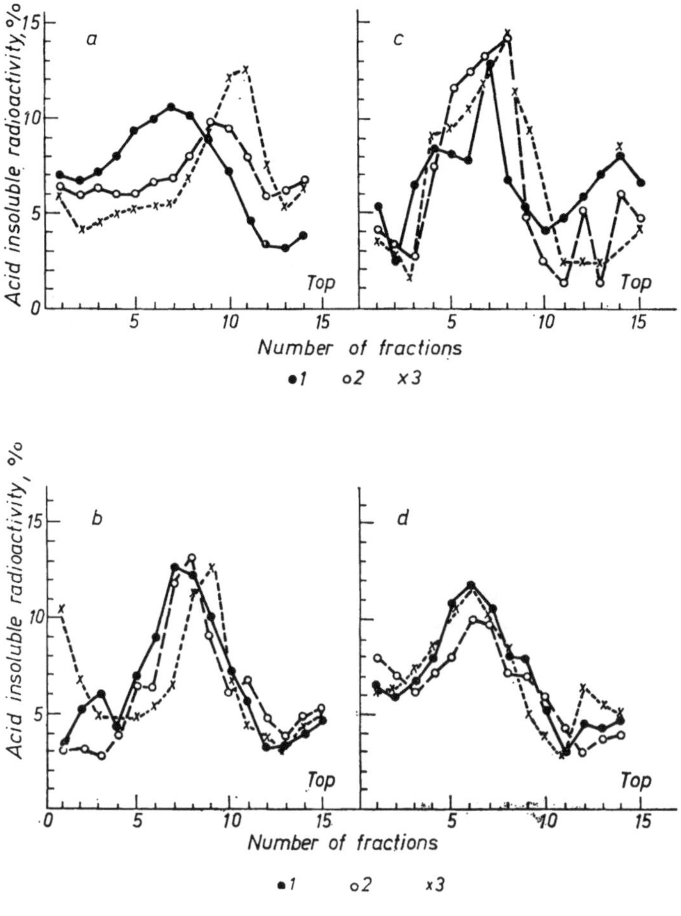

Fig. 5. Sedimentation profiles of pulse-labeled DNA from HeLa 2 h-63 cells treated with UV-light ($10\,J \cdot m^{-2}$, a); 7-bromomethyl-benz(a)anthracene (1 μg/ml, b), γ-rays (5 krad, c), 2-aminofluorene (10 μg/ml, d).
Caffeine (final concentration is 10^{-2} M) and ^{3}H-thymidine (13 Ci/mM; 20 μCi/ml) were added together to growth medium immediately after treatment for 60 min. The cells were lysed at the bottom of centrifuge tube in lysing solution containing 0.5 n NaOH with 1% sodium dodecylsulphate, 0.2% sodium deoxycholate and 0.05 M EDTA. 5-20% isokinetic alkaline sucrose gradient. Ultracentrifugation was performed in a rotor SW-65 of L2-65 Spinco centrifuge at 42000 rpm for 90 min at 20 °C. 1 — control; 2 — treatment; 3 — caffeine together with ^{3}H-thymidine after treatment (R. I. Pinto's, F. L. Vikhanskaya's and L. V. Olennikova's-data).

A more clear-cut relationship between the DNA repair at the molecular and cellular levels was established in experiments on cells from patients with Xeroderma pigmentosum. Clinically, biochemically and genetically, this hereditary disease due to somatic recessive mutation is not homogenous. Xeroderma pigmentosum may be caused by various molecular defects — failure of excision repair (CLEAVER, 1974), post-replication repair (LEHMANN et al. 1975), photoreactivation (SUTHERLAND et al. 1975) in UV-irradiated cells and disturbances in the repair of lesions induced by ionizing radiation, possibly as a consequence of deficient repair DNA polymerase (MIKHELSON et al., 1974).

Table 6. The effect of caffeine on survival, chromosome aberrations, and DNA repair in human and plant cells.

Cells	Criteria	Ionizing radiation	UV-light
HeLa Zh-63	Survival	+	+
	Unscheduled synthesis of DNA	+	+
	Repair of DNA single-strand breaks (SSB) in buffer, 1 krad	+	
	Repair of DNA SSB in growth medium, 20 krad	—	
	Repair of DNA double-strand breaks in growth medium, 20 krad	—	
	Post-replication repair of DNA (in cells pulse-labelled together with caffeine)		+
Peripheral blood lymphocytes	Chromosome aberrations, G_0-G_1	—	
	Chromosome aberrations, $S-G_2$	+	
	Unscheduled synthesis of DNA	+	+
	Repair of DNA SSB, 20 krad	+	
Buckwheat roots 2n	Chromosome aberrations	+	
4n	Chromosome aberrations	+	
Vicia faba, roots	Chromosome aberrations, G_1	—	
	Chromosome aberrations, G_2	+	
	Unscheduled synthesis of DNA	+	

\+ Survival decrease, chromosome aberrations increase, inhibition of DNA repair
— No effect

In our laboratory we studied processes of the DNA repair in lymphocytes of two patients with Xeroderma pigmentosum of a typical clinical picture but belonging to two different forms. In the first case (Xp I) cells are sensitive to UV-light only, while in the second (Xp II) they are sensitive to UV-light and ionizing radiation. The second form was first described in our laboratory by V. M. MIKHELSON and E. V. HAIKAZYAN (1972) and then was not detected by other investigators.

As a result of UV-irradiation a reduced level of the unscheduled synthesis of DNA and increased frequency of chromosome aberrations were revealed in peripheral blood lymphocytes of the both patients (Fig. 6).

By their sensitivity to ionizing radiation and ability to rejoin γ-ray-induced DNA single-strand breaks lymphocytes of patients with Xp I and Xp II vary considerably. In the case of Xp I unscheduled synthesis of DNA, frequence of chromosome aberrations and repair of DNA single-strand breaks did not differ any significantly from the same parameters in cells of a healthy man and phenotypically normal sister of the patient (despite the fact that unscheduled synthesis of DNA is delayed as compared to the control) (Fig. 7). In the case of Xp II the frequency of X-ray-induced chromosome aberrations is

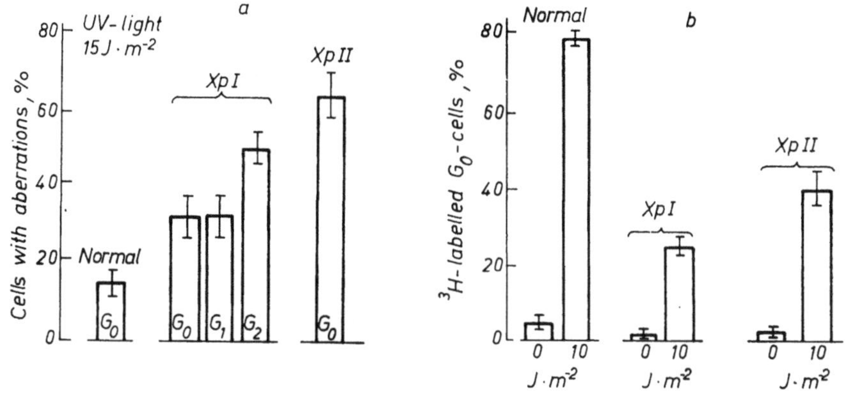

Fig. 6. Frequency of chromosome aberrations in PHA-stimulated (a) and unscheduled synthesis of DNA in non-stimulated (b) peripheral blood lymphocytes of healthy man (normal) and patients with Xeroderma pigmentosun (Xp) after UV-light-irradiation.

a. UV-light-irradiation immediately after (G_0), 18 h later — (G_1) and 48 h later — (G_2) PHA-treatment. Incubation in the medium for 54 h. Colchicine was added 4 h before fixation. Deletions, fragments, dicentrics and rings in metaphases were taken into account. For details see Mikhelson et al., 1974. (E. I. Genter's and I. S. Noskova's-data).

b. UV-light-irradiated cells were treated with ^{3}H-thymidine (13 Ci/mM; 10 μCi/ml) for 4 h. Emulsion of "P" type was exposed for 8 weeks at 4 °C. Cells containing 8—30 grains above the nucleus were taken into account. 500 cells were counted in each variant. For details see Genter, Noskova and Mikhelson, 1974.

increased, DNA unscheduled synthesis is weakened drastically and the repair of DNA single-strand breaks is lacking (Fig. 7, Table 7).

Consequently, in lymphocytes of patients suffering from Xeroderma pigmentosum there is a complete correlation between repair processes at the molecular and cellular levels. In the other words, results of experiments on higher eukaryotic cells in the case of a genetic defect are analogous to those carried out on bacteria. Keeping in mind that known DNA repair processes in microorganisms and higher eukaryots are similar in quality it can be said with confidence that DNA repair determines the reversibility of chromosome abnormalities and recovery of the viability in cells of higher organisms. The second conclusion from this common rule is that non-repaired lesions of DNA single-strand (and not only double-strand) breaks among them, can be the cause of chromosome aberrations and lethal effects after irradiation. The same conclusion was drawn by

Painter et al. (1976) who had analysed the reparability of DNA breaks in mammalian cells at the action of radioactive jodine. Such conclusion may seem trivial, but it must be remembered that there is a tendency to regard single-strand breaks as insignificant based on their role in the cell death (Lett et al. 1972; Fox and Fox 1974).

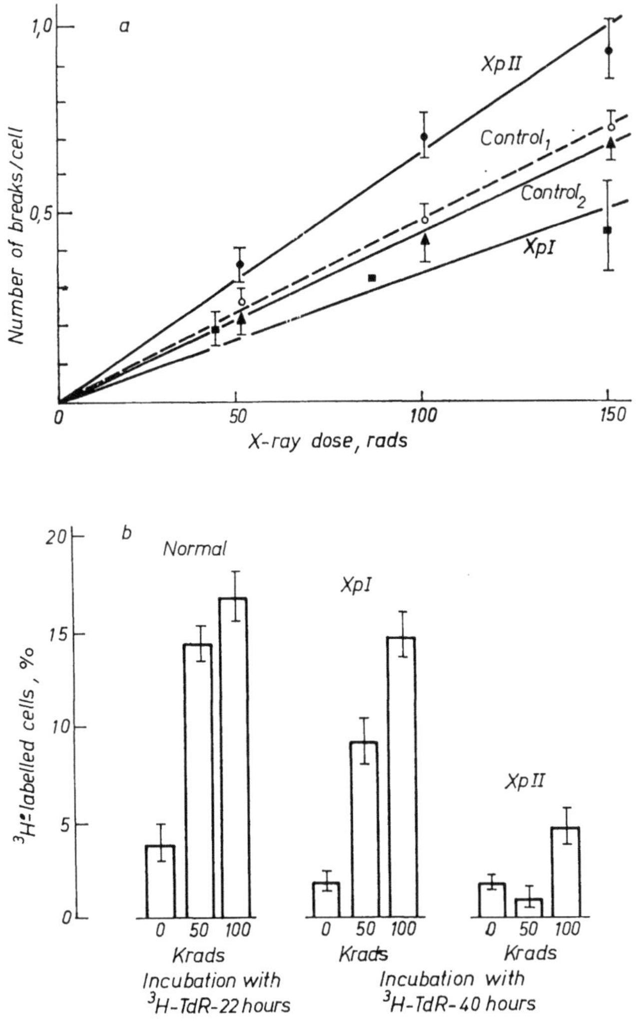

Fig. 7. Frequency of chromosome aberrations in X-ray-irradiated in G_0 stage PHA-stimulated (a) and unscheduled synthesis of DNA in γ-ray-irradiated non-stimulated peripheral blood lymphocytes in patients with two forms of Xeroderma pigmentosum (Xp), of a healthy man (control$_1$) and healthy sister of patient with Xp II (control$_2$).

a. X-ray-irradiation immediately after addition of PHA. For details see Mikhelson et al., 1974.

b. ^{3}H-thymidine was added to medium for 22 h or 40 h immediately after irradiation. For the rest details see legend to Fig. 6b (V. M. Mikhelson's, E. I. Genter's and E. I. Slonimskaya's-data).

Table 7. Frequency of chromosome aberrations and DNA repair in peripheral blood lymphocytes in Xeroderma pigmentosum patients

Kind of radiation	Criteria	Form	
		Xp I	Xp II
UV-light	Chromosome aberrations, G_0	Increased	Increased
	Chromosome aberrations, G_1 and G_2	Increased	Increased
	Unscheduled synthesis of DNA in non-stimulated cells (G_0)	Decreased	Decreased
X-rays and γ-rays	Chromosome aberrations, G_0	Normal	Increased
	Unscheduled synthesis of DNA, G_0	Normal (somewhat delayed)	Decreased
	Repair of DNA single-strand breaks	Normal	Absent

Conclusion

It would be possible to estimate the contribution of DNA repair to cell viability after irradiation only in cases when all manifestations of the activity of repair systems are blocked completely. Upon assumption that DNA repair plays the important role in maintenance of the viability of an intact cell (Paribok and Waldstein, 1970; Zhestyanikov, 1974), no absolute qualitative evaluation of such contribution is possible. Moreover, the DNA repair is a most essential but not the only factor that determines the cell radiosensitivity (Zhestyanikov, 1968). The cell death occurs at radiation doses after the action of which DNA breaks are fully repaired. The cause of radiation lethal effect, along with DNA structural defects, may be the respiratory failure (Swenson and Schenley, 1972) or the alteration of informational integrity (Rasmussen, Reisner and Painter, 1970; Brent and Wheatley, 1971). Experiments on *E. coli* cells carried out in our laboratory are an example of this idea (Zhestyanikov, Barenfeld and Barskaya, 1975).

The priming activity of DNA in RNA synthesis in vitro was investigated in *E. coli* B/r after exposure to X-rays and post-irradiation incubation in growth medium. It was found to be repaired completely only when cells had been irradiated with 9,3 krad. It recovered partially (about one third) at irradiation with 18,6 krad, the dose after which nearly all DNA single-strand breaks are repaired (a fraction of non-reparable double-strand breaks is about 0.1 of the whole number of single-strand breaks).

The existence of mutations blocking one or another of the repair mechanisms permit to estimate a relative contribution of an appropriate recovery system to elimination of lethal lesions in the cell. All the above shows that this can be done only on bacteria. Introduction into *E. coli* cells of mutations *uvr* A and *rec* A prevents completely the repair of UV-induced lesions. In double mutant *E. coli* K12 *uvr* A *rec* A one pyrimidine is one lethal hit, single *uvr* A mutant is able to tolerate 50-times more dimers, and the wild type — 3000 dimers per lethal hit (Howard-Flanders and Boyce, 1966). From this it follows that *uvr* A-dependent repair system eliminates about 98% of lethal lesions while the *rec* A-dependent system, the remaining 2% (Table 8).

Detection of three types of repair of X-ray-induced DNA single-strand breaks enables us to estimate a contribution of separate repair systems to elimination of these lesion

(TOWN, SMITH and KAPLAN, 1973). Ultrafast (radiochemical, non-enzymatic) repair, eliminates 25—75% of breaks after irradiation under aerobic or anoxic conditions. Fast repair, or DNA polymerase I-dependent repair, eliminates 70—20% of the breaks while slow repair eliminates the rest (Table 8). At the same time, the contribution of the repair of single-strand breaks and of the excision repair of bases modified by ionizing radiation to the survival of *E. coli* is not evaluated.

The contribution of various repair systems to recovery of the viability of mammalian cells injured by irradiation is not yet known.

Table 8. Contribution of DNA repair systems to the recovery of viability of bacteria and mammalian cells after irradiation

Radiation	Kind of DNA lesions	*Escherichia coli* Role in lethal effect	*Escherichia coli* Repair mechanism	Mammalian cells Role in lethal effect	Mammalian cells Repair mechanism
UV-light	Pyrimidine dimers of cyclobutane type	+	UvrAB dependent: 98% RecA-dependent: 2%*	+	Excision repair: + Post-replication repair (bypass of lesion and replication repair including): +
	Other photoproducts	?	?	Possible	?
Ionizing	Single-strand breaks	+	Non-enzymatic (ultrafast): 25% (O_2) 75% (N_2) PolA-dependent (fast): 70—75% (O_2) 15—20% (N_2) PolA-independent (slow): 5—10%**	+	Ultrafast — Fast + Slow +
	Double-strand breaks	+	—	+	+
	Alteration of bases	Possible	Excision repair: +	Possible	Excision repair: +

* HOWARD-FLANDERS and BOYCE, 1966

** TOWN, SMITH and KAPLAN, 1973; TOWN, 1975

References

[1] BACHMANN, B. I., LOW, K. B., TAYLOR, A. L.: Bacteriol. Revs. **40**, 116—167 (1976)

[1a] BRENT, T. P., WHEATLEY, G. A.: Intern. J. Rad. Biol. **19**, 339—348 (1971)

[2] BUHL, S. N., SETLOW, R. B., REGAN, J. D.: Biophys. J. **13**, 1265—1275 (1973)

[3] CLEAVER, J. E.: Adv. Radiat. Res. **4**, 1—75 (1974)

[4] CLARK, A. J., GANESAN, A.: 1975. In: Molecular Mechanisms for Repair of DNA, part B. (Eds: P. C. Hanawalt, R. B. Setlow), Plenum, 431—438.

[5] Clark, A. J.: Ann. Rev. Genetics **7**, 67—86 (1974)
[6] Fangman, W. L., Russel, M.: Molec. Gen. Genetics **110**, 332—347 (1971)
[7] Fox, B. W., Fox, M.: Intern. J. Radiat. Biol. **24**, 497—504 (1973)
[8] Genter, E. I., Noskova, I. S., Mikhelson V. M., 1974. In: Functional Morphology, Genetics and Biochemistry of the Cell, Nauka (Russian) Leningrad, 206—208
[9] German, J.: Progr. Med. Gent. **8**, 61—101 (1972)
[10] Hadi, S. M., Goldthwait, D. A.: Biochemistry **10**, 4986—4994 (1971)
[11] Haikazyan, E. V., Mikhelson, V. M., Zhestyanikov, V. D.: Cytology (Russian) **15**, 881—887 (1973)
[12] Haikazyan, E. V., Mikhelson, V. M., Zhestyanikov, V. D.: Cytology (Russian) **16**, 1135 — 1140 (1974)
[13] Hamilton, L. D., Mahler, I., Grossman L., 1975 In: Molecular Mechanisms for Repair of DNA, part A. (Eds: P. C. Hanawalt, R. B. Setlow), Plenum, 235—243
[14] Haynes, R. B., 1975. In: Molecular Mechanisms for Repair of DNA, part B. (Eds: P. C. Hanawalt, R. B. Setlow), Plenum, 529—540
[15] Heijneker, H. L.: Nucl. Acids Res. **2**, 2147—2161 (1975)
[16] Heijneker, H. L., Pennekock, H., Oosterbaan, R. A., Pouwels, P. H., Bron, S., Arwert, F., Venema, G.: Proc. Nat. Acad. Sci USA **68**, 2967—2971 (1971)
[17] Higgins, N. P., Kato, K., Strauss, B.: J. Molec. Biol. **101**, 417—425 (1976)
[18] Howard-Flanders, P., Boyce, R. P.: Radiat. Res. suppl. **6**, 154—184 (1966)
[19] Johnson, R. C., 1975. In: Molecular Mechanisms for Repair of DNA, part A. (Eds: P. C. Hanawalt. R. B. Setlow), Plenum, 325—325
[20] Kleijer, W. J., Hoeksema, J. L., Sluyter M. L., Bootsma, D.: Mutat. Res. **17**, 385—394 (1973)
[21] Körner, I., Malz, W.: Studia biophysica **41**, 11—20 (1973)
[22] Körner, I., Malz, W.: Studia biophysica **51**, 115—126 (1975)
[23] Körner, I., Malz, W., Günter, K.: Studia biophysica **47**, 127—136 (1974)
[24] Krupnova G. F., Alekhina, G. M., 1974. In: Functional Morphology, Genetics and Biochemistry of the Cell, Nauka (Russian), Leningrad, 214—216
[25] Krupnova, G. F., Seitkhozhaev, A. I.: Cytology (Russian) **16**, 1005—1009 (1974)
[26] Laipis, P. J., Ganesan, A. T.: Proc. Nat. Acad. Sci. USA **69**, 3211—3214 (1972)
[27] Lehmann, A. R.: Biophys. J. **12**, 1316—1325 (1972a)
[28] Lehmann, A. R.: J. Molec. Biol. **66**, 319—337 (1972b)
[29] Lehmann, A. R.: Life Sci. **15**, 2005—2016 (1974)
[30] Lehmann, A. R., Kirk-Bell, S.: Mutat. Res. **26**, 73—82 (1972)
[31] Lehmann, A. R., Kirk-Bell, S., Arlett, C. F., Paterson, M. C., Lohman, P. H. M., de Weerd-Kastelein, E. A., Bootsma, D.: Proc. Nat. Acad. Sci. USA **72**, 219—223 (1975)
[32] Lett, J. T., Sun, C., Wheeler, K. T., 1972. In: Molecular and Cellular Repair Processes. (Eds: R. F. Beers et al.) Johns Hopkins Univ. Press), Baltimore, 147—158
[33] Mazza, G., Fortunato, A., Ferrari, E., Canosi, U., Falaschi, A., Polsinelli, M.: Molec. Gen. Genetics **136**, 9—30 (1975)
[34] Mikhelson, V. M., Haikasyan, E. V.: Proc. Acad. Sci. USSR (Russian) **206**, **1462—1464** (**1972**)
[35] Mikhelson, V. M., Haikasyan, E. V., Genter, E. I., Pleskach N. M.: Cytology (Russian) **16**, 203—210 (1975)
[36] Painter, R. B., Young, B. R., Burki, H. J.: Proc. Nat. Acad. Sci. USA **71**, 4836—4838 (1974)
[37] Paribok, V. P., Waldstein, E. A., 1970. In: Postradiation Repair (Ed. V. P. Paribok), Atomizdat. Moscow, 314—335
[38] Paterson, M. C., Smith, B. P., 1976. Second Intern. Workshop an Repair Mechanisms in mammalian Cells, Noordwijkerhout, 32a.
[39] Pinto, R. I., Vikhanskaya, F. L., Falkovskaya, L. P., Semenova, E. G.: Proc. Acad. Sci. USSR (Russian) **214**, 691—693 (1974)

[40] Rasmussen, R. E., Reisner, B. L., Painter R. B.: Intern. J. Rad. Biol. **17**, 285—290 (1970)
[41] Robbins, J. H., Kraemer, K. H., Lutzner, M. A., Festoff, B. W., Coon, H. G.: Ann. Intern. Med. **80**, 221—248 (1974)
[42] Sedgwick, S. G., Bridges, B. A.: Molec. Gen. Genetics **119**, 93—102 (1972)
[43] Sedgwick, S. G., Bridges, B. A.: Nature **249**, 348—349 (1974)
[44] Sedliaková, M., Brosmanová, J., Slezariková, V., Mašek, F., Findlová, E.: Neoplasma **22**, 361—384 (1975)
[45] Semenova, E. G., Volkova, Z. M., Zhestyanikov, V. D.: Cytology (Russian) **16**, 1010—1015 (1974)
[46] Skavronskaya, A. G.: News Acad. Med. Sci. (Russian) N 12, 56—63 (1974)
[47] Small, G. D.: J. Bacteriol. **124**, 176—181 (1975)
[48] Smith, K. C.: In: Photophysiology (Ed. D. Giese) AP, **6**, 204—278 (1971)
[49] Sutherland, B. M., Rice, M., Wagner, E. K.: Proc. Nat. Acad. Sci. USA **72**, 103—107 (1975)
[50] Svetlova, M. P., Tomilin, N. V., Zhestyanikov, V. D.: Proc. Acad. Proc. Sci. USSR (Russian) **216**, 430—433 (1974)
[51] Svetlova, M. P., Tomilin, N. V., Savel'eva, G. E., Zhestyanikov, V. D., 1974. In: Functional Morphology, Genetics and Biochemistry of the Cell, Nauka (Russian), Leningrad, 178—180.
[52] Swenson, P. A., Schenley, R. L.: J. Bacteriol. **111**, 653—658 (1972)
[53] Tait, R. C., Harris, A. L., Smith, D. W.: Proc. Nat. Acad. Sci. USA **71**, 675—679 (1974)
[54] Tomilin, N. V.: Molec. Gen. Genetics **129**, 97—103 (1974a)
[55] Tomilin, N. V.: Molecular Biology (Russian) **8**, 557—568 (1974b)
[56] Tomilin, N. V.: Cytology (Russian) **19**, 1086—1109 (1977)
[57] Tomilin, N. V., Mosevitskaya, T. V.: Mutat. Res. **20**, 429—432 (1973)
[58] Tomilin, N. V., Mosevitskaya, T. V.: Mutat. Res. **27**, 147—156 (1975)
[59] Tomilin, N. V., Svetlova, M. P.: FEBS Letters **43**, 185—188 (1974)
[59a] Town, C. D., 1975. In: Proc. XI. Internat. Cancer Congr., **5**, 157—163 (Stockholm).
[60] Town, C. D., Smith, K. C., Kaplan, H.: Current Topics Radiat. Res., **8**, 351—399 (1973)
[61] Vikhanskaya, F. L., Pinto, R. I.: Proc. Acad. Sci. USSR (Russian) **226**, 1436—1439 (1976)
[62] Youngs, D. A., Smith, K. C.: Nature new Biol. **244**, 240—241 (1973)
[63] Zakharov, I. A., 1976. In: Physiological Genetics, Medicina. Leningrad, 114—160.
[64] Zherebtsov, S. V., Tomilin, N. V.: Biochim. et biophys. Acta **383**, 16—22 (1975)
[65] Zhestyanikov, V. D.: Nature **210**, 1231—1232 (1966)
[66] Zhestyanikov, V. D., 1968. Recovery and radioresistance of the cell. Nauka. Leningrad, 1—351.
[67] Zhestyanikov, V. D.: Studia biophysica **19**, 61—101 (1970)
[68] Zhestyanikov, V. D.: Radiobiology, Inform. Bull. (Russian) N 16, 5—10 (1974)
[69] Zhestyanikov, V. D.: Medical Radiology (Russian) N 1, 32—38 (1975)
[70] Zhestyanikov V. D., Barenfeld, L. S., Barskaya, T. V., 1975. In: Molecular Mechanisms for Repair of DNA, part B. (Eds: P. C. Hanawalt, R. B. Setlow), Plenum, N.Y., 497—500.
[71] Zhestyanikov, V. D., Savel'eva, G. E.: Proc. Acad. Sci. USSR (Russian) **226**, 1439—1442 (1976)
[72] Zhestyanikov, V. D., Semenova, E. G., Volkova, Z. M.: Cytology (Russian) **16**, 868—873 (1974)
[73] Zhestianikov, V. D., Svetlova, M. P., Tomilin, N. V., Savel'eva, G. E.: Studia biophysica **53**, 43—46 (1975)

The Biological Specificity of DNA Synthesis

CORNELIA SCHROEDER

Lehrstuhl Virologie der Charité, Humboldt-Universität zu Berlin, 104 Berlin, DDR

This paper is not meant as a review on DNA replication. Quite a few excellent reviews of this field have appeared recently (among others: SCHEKMAN et al., 1974; GEFTER, 1975; DRESSLER, 1975 and GEIDER, 1976) to which the reader is guided. Rather, this paper focuses on the question of biological specificity in processes of DNA synthesis, concentrating on the function of DNA polymerases.

Although DNA is chemically the same in all species (disregarding modifications for the moment), a biological specificity of DNA synthesis, documented by the presence of different DNA polymerases in different species and even within one cell, clearly exists. This specificity is expressed on different levels: First, the DNA polymerases of one cell are involved in different sub-processes of replication and alternative or exclusive repair pathways; second, in vivo they specifically replicate their "own" DNA; and third, they maintain a specific error rate during replication. Each of the following chapters is dedicated to one of these points.

Division of labour between DNA polymerases within the prokaryotic cell

Cellular organisms possess more than one, usually at least three independent DNA polymerases (but see LOOMIS et al., 1976). This is true for the bacteria where the pattern of DNA polymerases (termed I, II and III) seems to be conserved in evolutionary distant species like *E. coli* (GEFTER et al., 1971) and *B. subtilis* (GASS and COZZARELLI, 1973) but also for higher eukaryotes; though the DNA polymerases of eukaryotes (WEISSBACH, 1975) do not coincide with the prokaryote pattern.

Some properties of the three *E. coli* DNA polymerases have been arranged in the table. Polymerase I and III have been definitely associated with DNA replication and repair, while the role of polymerase II remains obscure, though it may partially substitute for the other two polymerases in their absence (TAIT and SMITH, 1974). DNA polymerase III is essential for replication (GEFTER et al., 1971 and NÜSSLEIN et al., 1971), it catalyzes the synthesis of OKAZAKI-pieces and may also take part in the final chromosome maturation step (TAIT and SMITH, 1974). Both these reactions may take place in or at membranes (TAIT and SMITH, 1974) which is reflected in the preference of a low ionic strength medium by purified DNA polymerase III (NÜSSLEIN et al., 1971, HEINZE and CARL, 1975). DNA polymerase I is involved in the degradation of RNA primers through its 5'—3' exonuclease function and in filling the resulting gaps between the OKAZAKI-pieces (OKAZAKI et al., 1971).

These steps are supposed to occur in the cytoplasm (TAIT and SMITH, 1974) and indeed, DNA polymerase I prefers a medium of relatively high ionic strength in vitro (the ionic strength requirements of several DNA polymerases are compared in GEIDER, 1976). Thus, the division of labour between the two DNA polymerases seems to be manifested in a compartmentation of the sub-processes they are responsible for.

DNA polymerase II has not proven essential for cell survival (CAMPBELL et al., 1972; HIROTA et al., 1972); however, the history of DNA polymerase I warns against hasty conclusions. After the discovery by DE LUCIA and CAIRNS in 1969 of the *pol*A (amber) mutants identifying the gene of DNA polymerase I which are viable in the "nonpermissive" host, it was generally supposed that DNA polymerase I is not essential for cell survival. Some plasmids, among them *col*E1 (GOEBEL, 1972), depend strictly on DNA polymerase I for replication. An analysis of *pol*A mutants by LEHMAN and CHIEN (1973) revealed that they induce a very low but detectable level of DNA polymerase I, estimated at 2—8 molecules per cell, while the levels of 5'—3' exonuclease were normal. By isolating temperature-sensitive 5'—3' exonuclease mutants, KONRAD and LEHMAN (1974) and OLIVERA and BONHOEFFER (1974) proved that at least this function of the DNA polymerase I is essential.

The division of labour between DNA polymerase I and III also extends into the realm of DNA repair. By and large, DNA polymerase I is a repair enzyme, and its contributions to DNA replication, primer excision and gap filling can also be viewed as a kind of repair. It is present at a 40-fold higher concentration than DNA polymerase III, reflecting the need for a constant high level of enzyme activity for repairing lesions which can occur at any time in the cell cycle. In contrast, the very low concentration of DNA polymerase III seems to be exactly fitted to the requirements of replication. The relation between the two polymerases is reminiscent of constitutive vs. inducible enzyme activity. I have mentioned above that the plasmid *col*E1 cannot replicate in *pol*A mutants (GOEBEL, 1972), although these mutants retain a residual polymerase I activity (LEHMAN and CHIEN, 1973). It is then difficult to understand how phages depending on DNA polymerase III for replication can manage with the 10 molecules usually present per uninfected cell. Thus, the question arises whether these phages (like λ and *phi*X 174) might be able to interfere with normal regulation in such a way that higher levels of DNA polymerase III are induced.

DNA polymerase I — negative mutants (*pol*A) replicate normally but exhibit a grossly repair-deficient phenotype including UV sensitivity and sensitivity towards MMS (DE LUCIA and CAIRNS, 1969). This could be interpreted to mean that the low residual activity of polymerase I (LEHMAN and CHIEN, 1973) is sufficient to maintain gap filling during DNA replication. However, despite this residual activity, double mutants *pol*A *rec*A are lethal for as yet unknown reasons (GROSS and GROSS, 1969). DNA polymerase I is certainly involved in the excision repair of UV lesions (DE LUCIA and CAIRNS, 1969; GROSS and GROSS, 1969; BOYLE et al., 1970). The 5'—3' exonuclease is able to degrade DNA containing pyrimidine dimers (KELLY et al., 1969), and the polymerase can fill the gaps.

Besides excision repair which is accurate, a type of post-replicational repair has been described (WITKIN, 1967) which is highly error prone and appears to be the source of UV-induced mutations. It involves DNA synthesis past non-coding (pyrimidine dimer) template regions (WITKIN, 1972), while none of the known DNA polymerases seems capable of such a reaction. In studies with *dna*E (DNA polymerase III) ts mutants the failure of such mutants to support error-prone repair at nonpermissive temperature has beeen taken to indicate a role of DNA polymerase III in this process (Bridges et al.,

1976) which again suggests that this enzyme might be inducible. Obviously, the requirements of error-prone repair are completely opposed to the requirements of normal DNA replication, and so if DNA polymerase III is actually involved, it will be in a different state and/or complex form than during replication synthesis.

Establishment of specificity in the replisome

It has been puzzling for a long time that DNA polymerases which when purified have similar catalytic properties and display no specificity whatsoever for their "own" DNA, should achieve such a marked specificity in vivo. In fact, the synthesis by purified DNA polymerases seems to be but a weak reflection of their capacity in vivo when complexed with other proteins.

This is quite logical since the basis of specificity is regulation: an "uncoupled" DNA polymerase must necessarily be rather inactive in order not to compete with the DNA synthesizing protein complex (called the replisome) for the DNA substrate. Only as a member of the replisome the DNA polymerase gains its full catalytic capacity. This applies to the true replication enzymes (DNA polymerase III, phage DNA polymerases) while the "repair" DNA polymerase I is probably not necessarily complexed in vivo though such complexes have been observed (HENDLER et al., 1975). This polymerase is capable of strand displacement itself, even as a fragment lacking 5′—3′ exonuclease activity (SETLOW et al., 1972) and, in agreement with its in this respect superior catalytic potency, requires less control in vivo.

The nature of the interactions between the various members of the replisome which adjust the replication polymerase to its function is hardly known, but great progress has been made in recent years by several groups in the reconstitution of active replisomes from their purified components (reviewed in SCHEKMAN et al., 1974 and GEIDER, 1976).

Why there should be a specificity for replicating "ones own" DNA is obvious: First, this is the chief weapon against the emergence of new viruses; without this specificity, the chances of conserving a large bacterial chromosome in an environment containing diverse episomal factors would be very low. Second, DNA replication must be exactly timed and adjusted to other cellular processes. Third, and this will be discussed below, the specificity achieved by the interactions within the replisome is expressed in the species-specific fidelity of DNA synthesis.

The decisive step during DNA synthesis ensuring the replication of homologous DNA and starting it off at the right moment in the cellular schedule is its initiation. The primary initiation step does not even require the presence of DNA polymerase; it can be viewed as a succession of steps beginning with the recognition of a certain DNA sequence, the origin of replication, by an initiation protein. This first step may be under negative control in the case of the replication of bacterial chromosomes and plasmids, and be released by the dilution or inactivation of a repressor in the course of the cell cycle (CABELLO et al., 1976), thus ensuring the presence of a small but defined number of plasmid DNA copies. In the case of bacteriophages survival depends on maximum offspring yields, and initiation frequency should not be under negative control (unless different phases of DNA replication have to be balanced). The next step may be the formation of an "initiation complex" around the initiation protein followed by the synthesis of the first RNA primer ("origin RNA"). The protein complex is then either re-

built or a new complex takes its place which then commences the synthesis of DNA. In this way initiation very effectively sets the replisome on the right track. How this can be achieved (and there may be a variety of ways) is illustrated by the following example:
The origin is often located in gene clusters specifying replication functions. Thus, the initiation of replication of the circular double stranded replicative form (RF) DNA of the phage *phi*X 174 is performed by the protein (endonuclease) coded for by geneA, the gene which also harbours the origin sequence (HENRY and KNIPPERS, 1974). This protein can only initiate replication of the RF by which it was coded (complementation is impossible) and is probably only functional as long as it is physically connected through ribosome, mRNA and RNA polymerase with its coding DNA. This mechanism secures an absolutely site-specific initiation.
As mentioned above, some bacteriophages depend on the host's DNA polymerase for replication and thus have overcome the specificity barrier. However, they do not use the host's replisome but a replisome containing host and phage factors which is assembled in a phage-specific initiation process (see reviews by SCHEKMAN et al., 1974 and GEIDER, 1976). The simplest case described so far has been the conversion of *E. coli* phage *G*4 single-stranded DNA to the double-stranded replicative form by three purified proteins of the host: the *dna*G product (a RNA polymerase) which synthesizes the primer, the DNA unwinding protein and DNA polymerase III (ZECHEL et al., 1975). Here specificity seems not to be due to the action of phage-specific proteins, but rather to the utmost simplicity of the system which is insufficient to perform any step in the host's DNA replication.
While initiation serves the purpose of forming the correct replisome at the right place and time, this does not explain all differences in quality between in vivo and in vitro DNA synthesis. Of all the replisomal constituents, the DNA binding proteins seem to have the strongest modifying effects on the DNA polymerase (most recently reviewed by GEIDER, 1976). Besides their function in initiation, DNA binding proteins have been found to bind to and activate DNA polymerase with a varying degree of specificity. While T4 DNA binding ("unwinding") protein does not activate the *E. coli* DNA polymerases II, and the *E. coli* DNA binding protein does not activate T4 DNA polymerase (SIGAL et al., 1972), phage T7 DNA polymerase can be activated by *E. coli* DNA binding protein (SCHERZINGER et al., 1973). When phage T4 DNA polymerase is complexed with its unwinding protein, it displays a 10—50 fold rate of polymerization (HUBERMAN et al., 1971) and a depressed 3′—5′ exonuclease activity (HUANG and LEHMAN, 1972), and gains the ability of strand displacement (NOSSAL, 1974). *E. coli* DNA polymerase I which, as mentioned above, is capable of strand displacement by itself, is probably not associated with an unwinding protein in vivo; it is actually inhibited by the *E. coli* unwinding protein (SIGAL et al., 1972).
A feature common to several replisomal entities described so far is the presence of proteins somehow linked to precursor synthesis. An outstanding example is the presence of deoxycytidinemonophosphate hydroxymethylase in the replisome of phage T4 (WOVCHA et al., 1973; TOMICH et al., 1974; CHE-SHEN CHIN et al., 1976). T4 DNA is exceptional in that the rare base hydroxymethylcytosine completely replaces cytosine (WYATT and COHEN, 1953) (rare base DNA also occurs in other phages, notably in those of *B. subtilis* (HEMPHILL and WHITELEY, 1975)), but T4 DNA polymerase cannot discriminate between dCTP and HMdCTP. Apparently, T4 DNA polymerase is "forced" to synthesize HMC-containing T4 DNA by the enzyme dCMP hydroxymethylase within the replisome.

Recently RICHARDSON and coworkers (MODRICH and RICHARDSON, 1975) found that the DNA polymerase of phage T7 is actually a complex of 2 proteins of which one is phage-coded but inactive without the other which turned out to be *E. coli* thioredoxin, a protein cofactor of E. *coli* ribonucleotide reductase (MARK and RICHARDSON, 1976). The involvement of enzymes of precursor synthesis indicates that deoxynucleotide triphosphates are produced within the replisome, and one might speculate that precursor synthesis at the replication fork constitutes an evolutionary advantage in a competetive situation between, for instance, different phages.

Maintenance of a species-specific error rate during replication

A very important aspect of specificity in DNA synthesis is its accuracy. The rate of spontaneous mutation is quite similar in most species, from the pro- to the eukaryotes (DRAKE, 1974). This means that while their DNA content has increased during evolution, the accuracy of replication (mutation rate per base pair replication) must have concomitantly improved (DRAKE, 1974).
The error rate of a DNA polymerase is influenced by its interactions with other proteins in the replisome, with the DNA and with metal ions.

Interactions within the replisome

The replication of phage λ depends on the host's DNA polymerase III in the lytic as well as in the lysogenic state. While the prophage λ is replicated by the *E. coli* replisome, free λ DNA replicates with a λ-specific replisome (see for instance review by GEIDER, 1976), and the mutation rate — although lastly determined by the same DNA polymerase — is 100 times higher in the lytic than in the integrated state (DOVE and FRANKLIN (1968), quoted in DOVE (1968)).
The involvement of phage T4 genes responsible for DNA replication in the determination of mutation rates has been thoroughly studied (reviewed by DRAKE (1973)) with mutator and antimutator mutants of these genes.
All replisomal proteins are coded by genes of this group (MORRIS et al., 1975, WOVCHA et al., 1973), and the protein interacting most strongly with T4 DNA polymerase, the DNA unwinding protein, also has the strongest effect on the accuracy of replication (besides the DNA polymerase itself).
It must be emphasized that a mutator phenotype displayed by a certain mutant does not prove the role of the affected gene in DNA replication. Many mutator genes specify repair functions, and the exact contributions of DNA replication and repair pathways to the spontaneous mutation rates have yet to be assessed. It is also important to distinguish between mutator genes and their gene products: Some of these genes may only be mutator genes in mutants where no functional gene product is synthesized and a more mutagenic pathway substitutes ("channeling", see VON BORSTEL and HASTINGS, 1976), while others are directly mutagenic by virtue of an altered gene product.
Purified mutator DNA polymerases are often less mutagenic than expected from in vivo mutation rates (HALL and LEHMAN, 1968). This means that the interactions within the replisome can amplify the inaccuracy (and thus probably in other cases also the accuracy) of the DNA polymerase.

Properties of purified DNA polymerases

Most work on the accuracy of purified DNA polymerases has been done with *E. coli* DNA polymerase I ((work on the catalytic functions of this enzyme until 1969 was reviewed by KORNBERG, 1969); TRAVAGLINI et al., 1975; SLOAN et al., 1975) with T4 DNA polymerase (among others HALL and LEHMAN, 1968; HERSHFIELD and NOSSAL, 1973d; MUZYCZKA et al., 1972; BESSMAN et al., 1974; and GOODMAN et al., 1974) and with the reverse transcriptase of AMV (SPRINGGALE et al., 1973, BATTULA and LOEB, 1975 and 1976; and SEAL and LOEB, 1976).
The fidelity of DNA synthesis cannot be explained alone by the formation of WATSON-CRICK hydrogen bonds between the incoming complementary deoxyribonucleotide triphosphate and the DNA template but rather is enforced by the enzyme, which discriminates between complementary and noncomplementary triphosphates and is able to excise noncomplementary nucleotides with its 3′—5′ exonuclease function. The recent work of LOEB and colleagues (TRAVAGLINI et al., 1975 and SLOAN et al., 1975) has elucidated that triphosphates are prealigned on the enzyme before polymerization and

Table. Properties of the DNA polymerases of *E. coli*

Polymerase / Gene	molecules per cell	speed of DNA synthesis in bases per min	associated nuclease activities	capable of strand displacement
I / *pol*A	400	50	3′—5′ 5′—3′	+
II / *pol*B	100	10	3′—5′	—
III / *pol*C	10	1000	3′—5′ 5′—3′ 1)	—

Polymerase / Gene	associated with DNA binding proteins	constituent of replisomes	essential for *E. coli* replication	involved in DNA repair	mutator gene	mutator enzyme
I / *pol*A	—	?	+ (5′—3′ exo)	+	+ 2)	?
II / *pol*B	+	?	—	+	+ 3)	?
III / *pol*C	+	+	+	+	+	+ 4)

1) LIVINGSTON et al., 1975
2) VACCARO and SIEGEL, 1975
3) MOSES, 1975
4) HALL and BRAMMAR, 1973
Most of the other data have been selected from GEFTER et al., 1972 and GEIDER, 1976.

that even in the absence of template the polymerase selects triphosphates with their sugar-base moiety in the same conformation as that in double helical DNA. Thus, orientational forces increase complementary and decrease noncomplementary nucleotide binding.

Once a noncomplementary nucleotide has been incorporated, it can be excised by the 3′—5′ exonuclease activity (found, up to now, in prokaryotic but not in eukaryotic DNA polymerases). This proofreading function specifically recognizes mispaired bases (Brutlag and Kornberg, 1972; Hershfield and Nossal, 1972) while it cannot remove dideoxythymidine monophosphate which pairs correctly from the 3′ terminus; the polymerase function, however, discriminates strongly against this analog (Atkinson et al., 1969).

Muzyczka et al. (1972) showed that the ratio of exonuclease to polymerase activity is enhanced in two antimutator and lowered in two mutator polymerases of phage T4. Another T4 mutator DNA polymerase nevertheless exhibited an increased nuclease to polymerase ratio, indicating that the inaccuracy of this mutant enzyme is due to an impaired specificity of the polymerase function, and not to a reduced proofreading ability (Hershfield and Nossal, 1973).

A study of the interactions between T4 DNA polymerase, intercalating drugs and DNA (Goodman et al., 1974b) has shed some light on the question of how replisomal proteins might interact with DNA polymerase to modify its accuracy. These drugs bind to and partially unwind DNA, thus modelling the effects of DNA binding proteins. Similar to these, they activate the DNA polymerase (at low drug concentrations; at higher concentrations they are inhibitory) and interfere with nuclease activity with the result of reducing the accuracy of DNA synthesis.

The role of the DNA template and of bivalent cations

The accuracy of replication depends not only on the replisome but also on the DNA template. Thus, the DNA polymerases of two closely related Bacillus species differing in the base composition of their DNA by 7% replicated homologous DNA more faithfully than the DNA of the other species (Stenesh and Roe, 1972). Geider (1976) suggested that *E. coli* DNA polymerase III is adapted to replicate single-stranded DNA free of secondary structure, while DNA polymerase I is adapted to replicate DNA sequences (initially covered by RNA primers) rich in secondary structure. This would explain the mutator phenotype of mutants lacking DNA polymerase I (Vaccaro and Siegel, 1975): in these mutants a polymerase less well adapted to secondary structure DNA has to fill the gaps between Okazaki-pieces and might, in doing so, be more error prone. A lot of evidence (quoted in Cox, 1972 and Presber et al., 1976) indicates that the accuracy of DNA synthesis has not only evolved in response to increasing genome size (Drake, 1974) but also in close interaction with the species-specific DNA base composition and its non-random distribution.

Finally, the role of metal ions remains to be discussed. Two metal ions are involved in the normal catalysis of DNA synthesis: Zinc ions are tightly bound to the polymerase's active site and serve to orient the 3′ OH end of the primer. Magnesium or manganous ions are required for binding the deoxynucleoside triphosphate to the polymerase (Mildvan, 1974). In most systems, manganous ions are mutagenic (among others T4

DNA polymerase: HALL and LEHMAN, 1968), however, one case has been described where magnesium ions reduce the accuracy of replication. This is the *M. luteus* DNA polymerase (LITMAN, 1971), and there may be a connection between the reversal of magnesium and manganous ion mutagenicity and the high GC content (72%) of the *M. luteus* DNA. Besides interacting with the triphosphates and the polymerases mutagenic metal ions can distort the DNA template which may then, in turn, alter the structure of the whole catalytic complex between the polymerase and its substrates. Finally there is the strong mutagenic effect of beryllium ions, which cannot, in contrast to manganous and other ions (SIROVER and LOEB, 1976) replace magnesium, but nevertheless strongly inhibit the 3'—5' exonuclease activity of *M. luteus* DNA polymerase (LUKE et al., 1975) relative to the polymerase activity, accompanied by an increased incorporation of noncomplementary nucleotides.

References

[1] ATKINSON, M. R., DEUTSCHER, M. P., KORNBERG, A., RUSSEL, A. F., MOFFAT, J. G.: Enzymatic synthesis of deoxyribonucleic acid XXXIV. Termination of chain growth by a 2',3'-dideoxyribonucleotide. Biochemistry **8**, 4897 (1969)

[2] BESSMAN, M. J., MUZYCZKA, N., GOODMAN, M. F., SCHNAAR, R.: Studies on the biochemical basis of spontaneous mutation II. The incorporation of a base and its analogue into DNA by wild type, mutator, and antimutator DNA polymerases. J. Molec. Biol. **88**, 409 (1974)

[3] BOYLE, J. M., PATERSON, M. C., SETLOW, R. B.: Excision repair properties of an *E. coli* mutant deficient in DNA polymerase. Nature **226**, 708 (1970)

[4] BRIDGES, B. A., MOTTERSHEAD, R. P., SEDGWICK, S. G.: Mutagenic DNA repair in *E. coli* III. Requirement for a function of DNA polymerase III in ultraviolet light mutagenesis. Mol. Gen. Genet. **144**, 53 (1976)

[5] BRUTLAG, D., KORNBERG, A.: Enzymatic synthesis of deoxyribonucleic acid XXXVI. A proofreading function for the 3'—5' exonuclease activity in deoxyribonucleic acid polymerases. J. Biol. Chem. **247**, 241 (1972)

[6] CABELLO, F., TIMMIS, K., COHEN, S. N.: Replication control in a composite plasmid constructed by in vitro linkage of two distinct replicons. Nature **259**, 285 (1976)

[7] CAMPBELL, J. L., SOLL, L., RICHARDSON, C. C.: Isolation and partial characterization of a mutant of *E. coli* deficient in DNA polymerase II. Proc. Nat. Acad. Sci., USA **69**, 2090 (1972)

[8] CHE-SHEN CHIU, TOMICH, P. K., GREENBERG, G. R.: Simultaneous initation of synthesis of bacteriophage T4 DNA and of deoxyribonucleotides. Proc. Nat. Acad. Sci., USA **73**, 757 (1976)

[9] COX, E. C.: On the organization of higher chromosomes. Nature New Biol. **239**, 133 (1972)

[10] DE LUCIA, P., CAIRNS, J.: Isolation of an *E. coli* strain with a mutation affecting DNA polymerase. Nature **224**, 1164 (1969)

[11] DOVE, W. F.: The genetics of the lambdoid phages. Ann. Rev. Genet. **2**, 305 (1968)

[12] DRAKE, J. W.: The genetic control of spontaneous and induced mutation rates in bacteriophage T4. Genetics **73** (Suppl.), 45 (1973)

[13] DRAKE, J. W.: Evolution in the microbial world. Symp. Soc. Gener. Microbiol. **XXIV**, 41 (1974)

[14] DRESSLER, D.: The recent excitement in the DNA growing point problem. Ann. Rev. Microbiol. **29**, 525 (1975)

[15] GASS, K. P., COZZARELLI, N. R.: Further genetic and enzymological characterization of the three *B. subtilis* deoxyribonucleic acid polymerases. J. Biol. Chem. **248**, 7688 (1973)

[16] GEFTER, M. L., HIROTA, Y., KORNBERG, T., WECHSLER, J. A., BARNOUX, C.: Analysis of DNA polymerases II and III in mutants of *E. coli* thermosensitive for DNA synthesis. Proc. Nat. Acad. Sci., USA **68**, 3150 (1971)

[17] GEFTER, M. L., KORNBERG, T., MOLINEUX, I. J., KHORANA, H. G., MENDICH, L., HIROTA, Y. (1972). Studies on DNA polymerases II and III of *E. coli.* DNA synthesis in vitro, R. D. Wells and R. B. Inman, eds., University Park Press, Baltimore, p. 71

[18] GEFTER, M. L.: DNA replication. Ann. Rev. Biochem. **44**, 45 (1975)

[19] GEIDER, K.: Molecular aspects of DNA replication in *E. coli* systems. Current Topics Microbiol. Immunol. **74**, 55 (1976)

[20] GOEBEL, W.: Replication of the DNA of the colicinogenic factor E1 (colE1) at the restrictive temperature in a DNA replication mutant temperature sensitive for DNA polymerase III. Nature New Biol. **237**, 67 (1972)

[21] GOODMAN, M. F., GORE, W. C., MUZYCZKA, N., BESSMAN, M. J.: Studies on the biochemical basis of spontaneous mutation III. Rate model for DNA polymerase-effected nucleotide misincorporation. J. Molec. Biol. **88**, 423 (1974a)

[22] GOODMAN, M. F., BESSMAN, M. J., BACHUR, N. R.: Adriamycin and daunorubicin inhibition of mutant T4 DNA polymerases. Proc. Nat. Acad. Sci., USA **71**, **1193** **(1974b)**

[23] GROSS, J. D., GROSS, M.: Genetic analysis of an *E. coli* strain with a mutation affecting DNA polymerase. Nature **224**, 1166 (1969)

[24] HALL, R. M., BRAMMAR, W. J.: Increased spontaneous mutation rates in mutants of *E. coli* with altered DNA polymerase III. Molec. Gen. Genet. **121**, 271 (1973)

[25] HALL, Z. W., LEHMAN, I. R.: An in vitro transversion by a mutationally altered T4 induced DNA polymerase. J. Molec. Biol. **36**, 321 (1968)

[26] HEINZE, J. E., CARL, P. L.: The effects of organic solvents on *E. coli* DNA polymerase III. Biochim. biophys. Acta **402**, 35 (1975)

[27] HEMPHILL, H. E., WHITELEY, H. R.: Bacteriophages of B. subtilis. Bacteriol. Rev. **39**, 257 (1975)

[28] HENDLER, R. W., PEREIRA, M., SCHARFF, R.: DNA synthesis involving a complexed form of DNA polymerase I in extracts of *E. coli.* Proc. Nat. Acad. Sci., USA **72**, 2099 (1975)

[29] HENRY, T. J., KNIPPERS, R.: Isolation and function of the gene A initiator of bacteriophage *phi*X 174, a highly specific endonuclease. Proc. Nat. Acad. Sci. USA **71**, 1549 (1974)

[30] HERSHFIELD, M. S., NOSSAL, N. G.: Hydrolysis of template and newly synthesized deoxyribonucleic acid by the 3′ to 5′ exonuclease activity of the T4 deoxyribonucleic acid polymerase. J. Biol. Chem. **247**, 3393 (1972)

[31] HERSHFIELD, M. S., NOSSAL, N. G.: In vitro characterization of a mutator T4 DNA polymerase. Genetics **73** (Suppl.), 131 (1973)

[32] HIROTA, Y., GEFTER, M., MENDICH, L.: A mutant of *E. coli* defective in DNA polymerase II activity. Proc. Nat. Acad. Sci., USA **69**, 3238 (1972)

[33] HUANG, WAI MUN, LEHMAN, I. R.: On the exonuclease activity of phage T4 deoxyribonucleic acid polymerase. J. Biol. Chem. **247**, 3139 (1972)

[34] HUBERMAN, J. A., KORNBERG, A., ALBERTS, B. M.: Stimulation of T4 bacteriophage DNA polymerase by the protein product of T4 gene 32. J. Molec. Biol. **62**, 39 (1971)

[35] KELLY, R. B., ATKINSON, M. R., HUBERMAN, J. A., KORNBERG, A.: Excision of thymine dimers and other mismatched sequences by DNA polymerase of *E. coli.* Nature **224**, 495 (1969)

[36] KONRAD, E. B., LEHMAN, I. R.: A conditional lethal mutant of *E. coli* K12 defective in the 5′—3′ exonuclease associated with DNA polymerase I. Proc. Nat. Acad. Sci., USA **71**, 2048 (1974)

[37] KORNBERG, A.: Active center of DNA polymerase. Science **163**, 1410 (1969)

[38] LEHMAN, I. R., CHIEN, J.: Persistence of DNA polymerase I and its 5′—3′ exonuclease activity in *pol*A mutants of *E. coli* K12. J. Biol. Chem. **248**, 7717 (1973)

[39] LITMAN, R. M.: The differential effect of magnesium and manganese ions on the synthesis of *poly* (dG · dC) and *M. luteus* DNA by *M. luteus* DNA polymerase. J. Molec. Biol. **61**, 1 (1971)

[40] Loomis, L. W., Rossomando, E. F., Chang, L. M. S.: DNA polymerase of *Dyctiostelium discoideum*. Biochim. biophys. Acta. **425**, 469 (1976)
[41] Luke, M. Z., Hamilton, L., Hollocher, T. C.: Beryllium-induced misincorporation by a DNA polymerase: A possible factor in beryllium toxicity. Biochem. biophys. Res. Commun. **62**, 497 (1975)
[42] Mark, D. F., Richardson, C. C.: *E. coli* thioredoscin: A subunit of bacteriophage T7 DNA polymerase. Proc. Nat. Acad. Sci., USA **73**, 780 (1976)
[43] Mildvan, A. S.,: Mechanism of enzyme action. Ann. Rev. Biochem. **43**, 357 (1974)
[44] Modrich, P., Richardson, C. C.: Bacteriophage T7 deoxyribonucleic acid replication in vitro. Bacteriophage T7 DNA polymerase: An enzyme composed of phage and host-specified subunits. J. Biol. Chem. **250**, 5515 (1975)
[45] Morris, C. F., Sinha, N. K., Alberts, B. M.: Reconstruction of bacteriophage T4 DNA replication apparatus from purified components: Rolling circle replication following *de novo* chain initiation on a single stranded circular DNA template. Proc. Nat. Acad. Sci., USA **72**, 4800 (1975)
[46] Moses, R. E.: DNA polymerase II of *E. coli*. Conference on eukaryotic DNA polymerases (Abstracts). Asilomar Conference Center, Monterey (1975)
[47] Muzyczka, N., Poland, R. L., Bessman, M. J.: Studies on the biochemical basis of spontaneous mutation I. A comparison of the deoxyribonucleic acid polymerases of mutator, antimutator, and wild type strains of bacteriophage T4. J. Biol. Chem. **247**, 7116 (1972)
[48] Nossal, N. G.: DNA synthesis on a double-stranded DNA template by the T4 bacteriophage DNA polymerase and the gene 32 unwinding protein. J. Biol. Chem. **249**, 5668 (1974)
[49] Nüsslein, V., Otto, B., Bonhoeffer, F., Schaller, H.: Function of DNA polymerase III in DNA replication. Nature New Biol. **234**, 285 (1971)
[50] Okazaki, R., Arisawa, M., Sugino, A.: Slow joining of newly replicated DNA chains in DNA polymerase I — deficient *E. coli* mutants. Proc. Nat. Acad. Sci., USA **68**, 2954 (1971)
[51] Olivera, B. M., Bonhoeffer, F.: Replication of *E. coli* requires DNA polymerase I. Nature **250**, 513 (1974)
[52] Presber, W., Schroeder, C., Krüger, D.: The evolution of mutation rates via DNA base composition and mutator genes: a proposition. J. Theor. Biol **59**, 353 (1976)
[53] Schekman, R., Weiner, A., Kornberg, A.: Multienzyme systems of DNA replication. Science **186**, 987 (1974)
[54] Setlow, P., Brutlag, D., Kornberg, A.: DNA polymerase: two distinct enzymes in one polypeptide. I. A proteolytic fragment containing the polymerase and 3′—5′ exonuclease functions. J. Biol. Chem. **247**, 224 (1974)
[55] Sigal, N., Delius, H., Kornberg, T., Gefter, M. L., Alberts, B. M.: A DNA unwinding protein isolated from *E. coli*: Its interaction with DNA and with DNA polymerases. Proc. Nat. Acad. Sci., USA **69**, 3537 (1972)
[56] Sirover, M. A., Loeb, L. A.: Metal activation of DNA synthesis. Biochem. biophys. Res. Commun. **70**, 812 (1976)
[57] Sloan, D. L., Loeb, L. A., Mildvan, A. S., Feldman, R. C.: Conformation of deoxynucleotide triphosphate substrates on DNA polymerase I from *E. coli* as determined by nuclear magnetic relaxation. J. Biol. Chem. **250**, 8913 (1975)
[58] Stenesh, J., Roe, B. A.: DNA polymerase from mesophilic and thermophilic bacteria II. Temperature dependence of nearest neighbour frequencies of the product from the DNA polymerase reaction. Biochem. biophys. Acta **272**, 167 (1972)
[59] Tait, R. C., Smith, D. W.: Roles for *E. coli* DNA polymerases I, II, III in DNA replication. Nature **249**, 5453 (1974)
[60] Tomich, P. K., Che-Shen Chiu, Wovcha, M. G., Greenberg, G. R.: Evidence for a complex regulating the in vitro activities of early enzymes induced by bacteriophage T4. J. Biol. Chem. **249**, 13 (1974)

[61] Vaccaro, K. K., Siegel, E. C.: Increased spontaneous reversion of certain frameshift mutations in DNA polymerase I deficient strains of *E. coli*. Molec. Gen. Genet. **141**, 251 (1975)

[62] von Borstel, R. C., Hastings, P. J. (1976). Mutagenic repair pathways in yeast. Proc. VII Intern. Congr. Photobiol. (Rome, Italy, 1976)

[63] Weissbach, A.: Vertebrate DNA polymerases. Cell **5**, 101 (1975)

[64] Witkin, E. M.: Mutation-proof and mutation-prone modes of survival in derivatives of *E. coli* B differing in sensitivity to ultraviolet light. Brookhaven Symp. Biol. **20**, 17 (1967)

[65] Witkin, E. M.: Ultraviolet light mutagenesis in repair deficient derivatives of *E. coli* B/r: *uvr*A*rec*B and *uvr*A*rec*C strains. Mutation Res. **16**, 235 (1972)

[66] Wovcha, M. G., Tomich, P. K., Che-Shen Chiu, Greenberg, G. R.: Direct participation of dCMP hydroxymethylase in synthesis of bacteriophage T4 DNA. Proc. Nat. Acad. Sci., USA **70**, 2196 (1973)

[67] Wyatt, G. R., Cohen, S. S.: The bases of the nucleic acids of some bacterial and animal viruses: the occurrence of 5-hydroxymethyl cytosine. Biochem. J. **55**, 774 (1953)

[68] Zechel, K., Bouché, J., Kornberg, A.: Replication of phage G4. IX. Novel and simple system for initiation of DNA synthesis. J. Biol. Chem. **250**, 4084 (1975)

[69] Livingston, D. M., Hinkle, D. C., Richardson, C. C.: Deoxyribonucleic acid polymerase III of Escherichia coli. Characterization of associated exonuclease activities. J. Biol. Chem. **250**, 470 (1975)

DNA REPAIR AFTER UV-IRRADIATION AND ALKYLATING AGENTS

Rejoining of Incision Breaks in the DNA of Ultraviolet- Irradiated *Proteus Mirabilis* Wildtype and UV-sensitive Mutants

K. Störl

Akademie der Wissenschaften der DDR
Forschungszentrum für Molekularbiologie und Medizin
Zentralinstitut für Mikrobiologie und experimentelle Therapie,
DDR-69 Jena, Beuthenbergstr. 11

1. Introduction

Single-strand breaks are introduced enzymatically in the DNA of UV-irradiated cells of *E. coli* as first step in the excision repair of photochemical lesions. As enzymatic repair proceeds, the lesions are excised and the resultant gaps are filled by the reaction of DNA-polymerase. Finally, the joining of the repaired fragments to the parental DNA strands occurs (Howard-Flanders, 1968).

The phenomenological analysis of repair defective mutants of *P. mirabilis* has indicated the existence of similar repair mechanisms in *P. mirabilis* as described for *E. coli* (Böhme, 1970). We investigated in a previous paper the excision capability for UV-induced pyrimidine dimers in different UV-sensitive strains of *P. mirabilis* (Störl, Mund and Venner, 1973) and found for UV-sensitive mutants with EXR- or REC-phenotype only a slightly lower excision ability in comparison to the wildtype. On the contrary HCR-mutants were not able to excise pyrimidine dimers.

For further study of the excision repair process after UV-irradiation in *P. mirabilis* we analyzed the appearance and rejoining of single-strand breaks in the DNA observed by sedimentation analysis in alkaline sucrose gradients.

In this connection we also examined the size of the DNA newly synthesized after UV-irradiation in *P. mirabilis* wildtype and HCR-mutants.

2. Materials and methods

The studies were carried out on the following bacteria:

P. mirabilis PG 273 (thr⁻) and PG 758 (thr⁻, arg⁻) as UV-resistant wildtype strains, PG 686 (HCR), PG 698 (REC) and PG 699 (EXR) as UV-sensitive mutants. All strains were isolated in the laboratory of Prof. Böhme (Gatersleben). For comparison *E. coli* K12 AB 1557 was used.

Cultivation conditions, UV-irradiation, sucrose gradient sedimentation, estimation of average molecular weights and single-strand breaks were already described (Störl and Mund, 1977).

3. Results and discussion

Ultraviolet irradiation of UV-resistant wildtypes of *P. mirabilis* results in a decrease of the molecular weight of single stranded DNA after a short time of incubation, indicating that single-strand breaks were introduced in the DNA during the first step of excision repair process (Störl and Mund, 1977). The number of single-strand breaks produced in the DNA depends on the UV-dose (Fig. 1).

The low number of breaks observed by sedimentation in alkaline sucrose gradients in comparison to the high number of single-strand breaks expected from dimer excision is an indication for the high repair capacity of the cells. The greater part of the excision-induced breaks must be repaired as fast as they are formed.

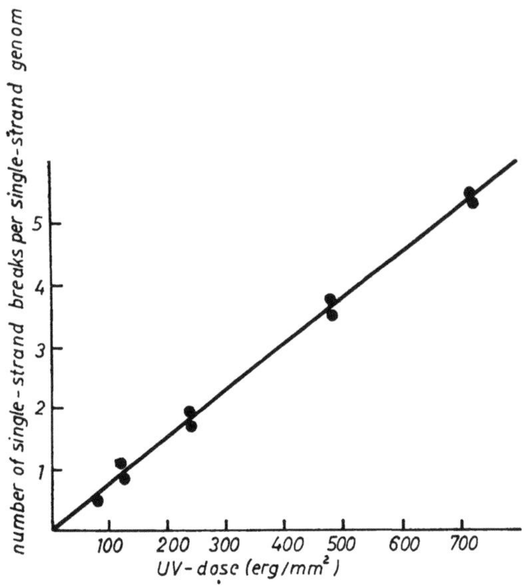

Fig. 1. Number of single-strand breaks induced in the DNA of PG 273 after irradiation with different UV-doses followed by 10 min incubation in minimal medium.

In Tab. 1 the number of single-strand breaks appearing immediately after UV-irradiation is represented with different strains of *P. mirabilis*.

The shift in the molecular weight of the DNA of REC- and EXR-mutants was similar to the wildtype. Probably the excision repair in these strains is also so effective that single-strand breaks induced can be repaired quickly at low UV-doses.

It is interesting to note that HCR-mutants of *P. mirabilis* which are deficient in excision of pyrimidine dimers (Störl, Mund and Venner, 1973) introduce single-strand breaks in their DNA immediately after UV-irradiation. In contrast to HCR-mutants of *E. coli*

Table 1. Appearance of incision breaks in the DNA of UV-sensitive mutants of *P. mirabilis* after irradiation with 80 erg/mm² and 10 min incubation in minimal medium.

Strains	Number of single-strand breaks/ single strand genom
PG 273 (wildtype)	0.15
PG 758 (wildtype)	0.20
PG 698 (REC)	0.80
PG 699 (EXR)	0.45
PG 686 (HCR)	2.0

(e.g. *E. coli* K12 AB 1886, which we have investigated for comparison) HCR-mutants of *P. mirabilis* appear not to be inhibited completely in incision step.
Furthermore, we have examined the completion of excision repair by investigation of the ability to rejoin the DNA-single-strand breaks during a longer time of incubation. Changes in the number of single-strand breaks were also estimated by sedimentation analysis of the corresponding DNA in alkaline sucrose gradients. After successful finishing of the excision repair process the single strand length of the DNA should return to the control value. The ability to rejoin single-strand breaks in course of the repair process depends on the UV-dose. After irradiation of *P. mirabilis* wildtype with UV-doses higher than ~240 erg/mm² complete repair did not occur. The behaviour of different strains of *P. mirabilis* after irradiation with relatively low UV-doses is shown in Fig. 2.

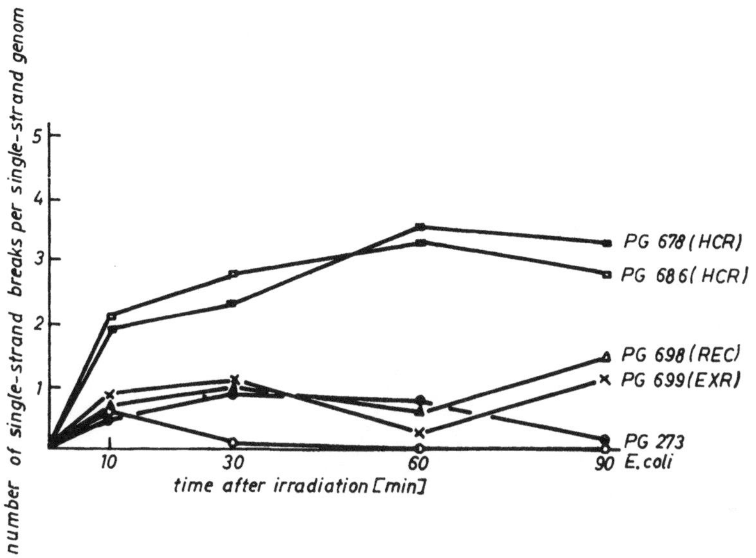

Fig. 2. Behaviour of incision breaks in the DNA of different UV-sensitive strains of *P. mirabilis* and *E. coli* K12 (AB 1157) in dependence of the time of post-irradiation incubation (UV-dose: 80 erg/mm²).

In *P. mirabilis* wildtype the repair is approximately complete after 90 min of incubation. However, the rejoining of single-strand breaks seems to be a little more effective in *E. coli* K12. On the contrary, HCR-mutants are not able to rejoin the single-strand breaks introduced in the DNA at the beginning of the repair process. They have only a low capacity to accomplish repair steps following incision.
REC- and EXR-strains were able to rejoin most of the induced single-strand breaks after irradiation with low UV-doses. The highest single-strand length of the DNA REC- and EXR-mutants approach 60 min. after irradiation. At this time the number of single-strand breaks remaining open was only a little higher than in the wildtype. After longer incubation times the number of single-strand breaks increases again. The large amount of DNA-degradation observed with REC-mutants after UV-irradiation complicates the interpretation of these results.
We have also looked at the DNA newly synthesized at the DNA containing pyrimidine

dimers. Changes in the parental (template) DNA, due to excision of pyrimidine dimers, may be observed as changes in the sedimentation rate of the newly synthesized DNA (daughter), because during replication gaps appear in this daughter DNA opposite to each dimer (Rupp and Howard-Flanders, 1968). Progress in the excision repair is reflected in an increase of the molecular weight of the DNA newly synthesized during longer incubation after UV-irradiation.

The sedimentation profiles in Fig. 3 show that in the wildtype of *P. mirabilis* immediately after irradiation a low-molecular weight, discontinous DNA is synthesized. With longer incubation times the size of the newly synthesized DNA increases and approximates the size of the nonirradiated control DNA, indicating that most of the pyrimi-

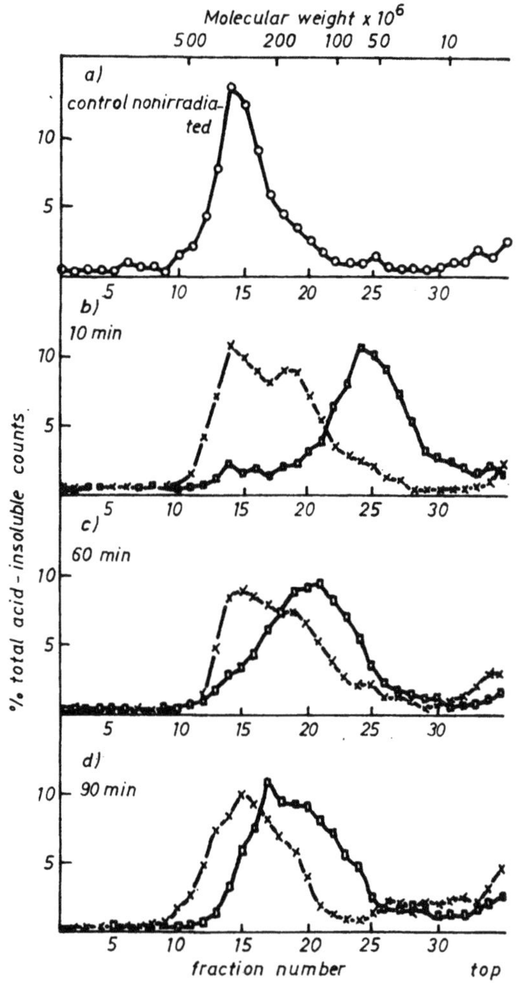

Fig. 3. Sedimentation profiles in alkaline sucrose gradients of parental (^{14}C-thymidine labelled) and newly synthesized daughter DNA (^{3}H-thymidine-pulse labelled) in *P. mirabilis* PG 273 (wildtype) after irradiation with 120 erg/mm² followed by different incubation times in minimal medium; × — × parental DNA, □ — □ daughter DNA.

dine dimers have been removed from the parental DNA. REC- and EXR-strains showed a similar behaviour as the wildtype at low UV-doses.
As can be seen in Fig. 4 the size of the DNA synthesized a short time after UV-irradiation in HCR-mutants was of very low molecular weight. The maintenance of this low-molecular weight, discontinous DNA also after longer incubation times corresponds with the incapability of HCR-mutants of *P. mirabilis* to excise pyrimidine dimers from the parental template strand.

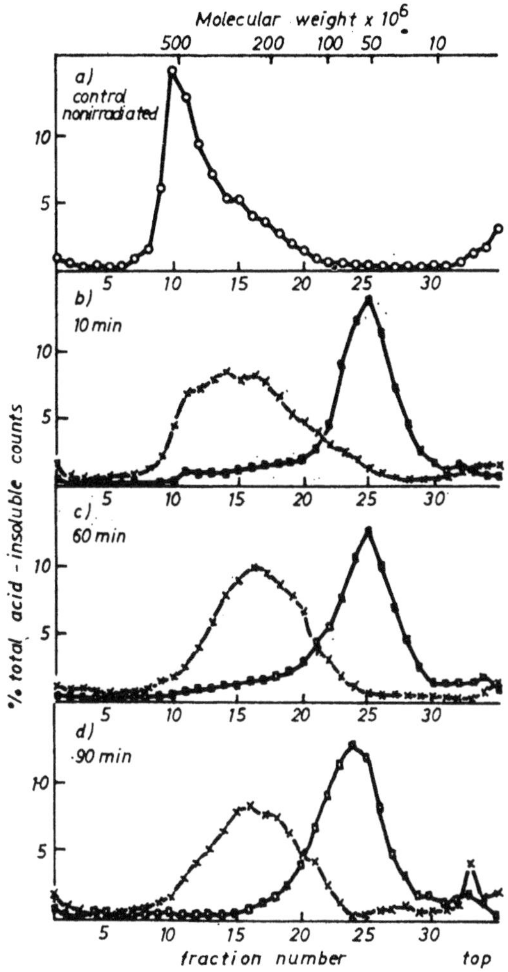

Fig. 4. Sedimentation profiles in alkaline sucrose gradients of parental (^{14}C-thymidine labelled) and newly synthesized daughter DNA (^{3}H-thymidine-pulse labelled) in PG 686 (HCR) after irradiation with 80 erg/mm². × — × parental DNA, □ — □ daughter DNA.

Summary

The appearance of single-strand breaks in the DNA of *P. mirabilis* wildtype and different repair defective mutants at the beginning of excision repair and their rejoining after dimer excision and completion of repair synthesis were studied by use of the alkaline sucrose gradients technique. The behaviour of REC- and EXR-mutants was similar to the wildtype at low UV-doses. Most of the single-strand breaks produced in the DNA immediately after UV-irradiation were rejoined during further incubation. On the contrary, HCR-mutants were not able to rejoin the single-strand breaks induced by the repair process.

References

[1] Böhme, H.: Studia biophysica **19**, 159—162 (1970)
[2] Howard-Flanders, P.: Annu. Rev. Biochem. **37**, 175—200 (1968)
[3] Rupp, W. D., Howard-Flanders, P.: J. Mol. Biol. **31**, 291—304 (1968)
[4] Störl, K., Mund, Ch., Venner, H.: Molec. gen. Genet. **124**, 259—268 (1973)
[5] Störl, K., Mund, Ch., 1977, Studia biophysica **61**, 231—243

UV-light Sensitivity and Split-dose Effects in two Strains of Murine Leukaemic L5178Y Cells

M. Walicka and J. Z. Beer

Department of Radiobiology and Health Protection, Institute of Nuclear Research, PL-03-195 Warszawa — Żerań

1. Introduction

In contrast to very extensive studies on effects of fractionation of X-ray doses, the effects of UV-light fractionation have been less investigated in mammalian cell systems. Han, Miletić and Petrović (1964), and Domon and Rauth (1973) studied these effects using murine L-cells. Various strains of Chinese hamster cells were used by Todd, Coohill, Helewell and Mahoney (1969), Humphrey, Sedita and Meyn (1970), Humphrey and Meyn (1972), and Thilly and Heidelberger (1973). Todd (1973) investigated effects of split doses of UV-light using human M-13 cells and Chinese hamster V7979 cells. Of all these authors, only Humphrey et al reported a correlation between sparing effect of UV-dose fractionation and UV-sensitivity of the two examined cell lines: they found that this effect occurred in a more UV-resistant cell line, whereas it could not be demonstrated in a more sensitive one.

In this paper we will describe another example of such a correlation found for two strains of murine leukaemic lymphoblasts: L5178Y-R and L5178Y-S and we shall describe observations which indicate that UV-light sensitivity at least to a certain exent depends on the ability to repair the UV-induced sublethal lesions.

2. Experimental

2.1. *Cell lines and cultivation*

Two strains of murine leukaemic lymphoblasts L5178Y (Fischer 1957) differing in their X-ray sensitivities by a factor of ca. 2 (Alexander and Mikulski 1961, Beer, Lett and Alexander 1963) were used in the experiments. Recently determined parameters characterizing their X-ray sensitivities are for L5178Y-R cells: $D_0 = 96$ rad, $D_q = 46$ rad, $n = 1.6$ and for L5178Y-S cells: $D_0 = 56$ rad, $D_q = 43$ rad, $n = 2.1$ (Walicka 1975).

L5178Y-R and L5178Y-S cells differ also in their UV-light sensitivity, the latter being more UV-light resistant. Thus the two cell strains are cross-sensitive to X-rays and UV-light (Beer, Szumiel and Walicka 1973 a, b, Walicka 1975). Parameters characterizing UV-light sensitivity of the strains used in the present studies will be given under 3.1.

A number of L5178Y cell strains differing in X-ray sensitivities have been used in various laboratories (e.g. Courtenay 1969, Fox and Fox 1973). The strains used by us are comparable with those designated by Lett, Parkins, Alexander and Ormerod (1964), and Lett and Alexander (1965) as R/F and S/F.

L5178Y-R cells transform spontaneously into L5178Y-S cells after several month of cultivation in vitro. For this reason maintenance of L5178Y-R cells requires alternate passages in vitro and in vivo. Both cell lines can be grown in vivo in DBA/2 mice. Inoculated intraperitoneally L5178-R cells produce ascitic tumours, whereas L5178Y-S cells tend to form solid tumours.
Mean diameters are 14 μm for L5178Y-R and 16 μm for L5178Y-S cells.
Cell cycle parameters for L5178Y-R cells have not been determined. For L5178Y-S cells they are: $G1 = 1.3$ h, $S = 6.4$ h, $G2 = 2.6$ h, $M = 0.5$ h (BEER, BOCIAN, BUDZICKA, ZIEMBA-ŻAK, KOPEĆ 1974).
Both cell lines were cultivated as suspensions in the FISCHER-medium (FISCHER, SARTORELLI 1964) containing 8% of calf serum (supplied by PAŃSTWOWA, WYTWÓRNIA, SUROWIC i SZCZEPIONEK, Lublin, Poland) and supplemented with 0.1 g/l of neomycin. Cell density was maintained in the range from 5×10^4 to 7×10^5 cells/ml for L5178Y-R strain, and from 23×10^3 to 7×10^5 cells/ml for L5178Y-S strain. Under these conditions mean doubling times varied from 14 to 15 h for L5178Y-R cells, and from 10.5 to 11.5 h for L5178Y-S cells.
Cell population densities were determined microscopically using a Bürker haemocytometer.

2.2. *Viability determination*

Viability of the cell cultures was determined by nigrosine staining (PAUL 1960).

2.3. *UV irradiation*

Germicidal làmp, type TUV-30 Philips (Eidhoven, The Netherlands) was used as a source of UV-light. This lamp emits approx. 90% of 254 nm UV-light. The lamp was equipped with a quartz jacket containing saturated aqueous sodium acetate solution to absorb ionizing components of the mercury vapour radiation.
Suspensions of 10^6 cells, unless otherwise stated in 5 ml of FISCHER-medium, were irradiated in 45 cm long quartz tubes placed horizontally, parallelly to the axis of the lamp. In some cases the cells were irradiated in the HANKS-solution without phenol red. In these experiments, before exposure, suspensions of the cells in the FISCHER-medium were centrifuged at 500 g and the cells were resuspended in the HANKS-solution. Immediately after irradiation the cells were placed back in the FISCHER-medium. If thereafter a second dose was to be applied, again before the exposure cells were transferred into the HANKS-solution. Unless otherwise stated, the cells were incubated between the doses at 37 °C.
Maximal thickness of the cell suspension layer was 2 mm. Absorption of 254 nm UV-light in various solutions and suspensions used in the experiments have been determined and the results are given in Table 1.
Mean exposure rate at a distance of 100 cm from the lamp, determined by uridine actinometry according to Shugar (1966), was 9.84 ± 0.37 (95% confidence interval) erg/mm² sec. For convenience we shall use the term "dose" for the product of so determined exposure rate and irradiation time, uncorrected for absorption.

Table 1. Absorption of 254 nm UV-light in 2 mm-thick layers of solutions and suspensions used in the experiments.

Absorbing layer	Absorption %
HANKS-solution without phenol red	0
15×10^4 L5178Y-R cells per ml in the HANKS-solution without phenol red	8
18×10^4 L5178Y-S cells per ml in the HANKS-solution without phenol red	13
FISCHER-medium	92
2×10^5 L5178Y-S cells per ml in the FISCHER-medium	94

2.4. *Survival determination*

Growth of L5178Y cells exposed to UV-light can be stimulated at later post-irradiation stages (WALICKA and BEER 1973, Fig. 1). For this reason estimations of survival of both strains used, on the basis of their growth observations were made by the backward extrapolation method of ALEXANDER and MIKULSKI (1960) modified as follows.
After irradiation, viability of the cell populations was determined by nigrosine staining at the times of cell counting. The cell counts taken at 1—2 day intervals were converted into relative cell numbers (Fig. 1).

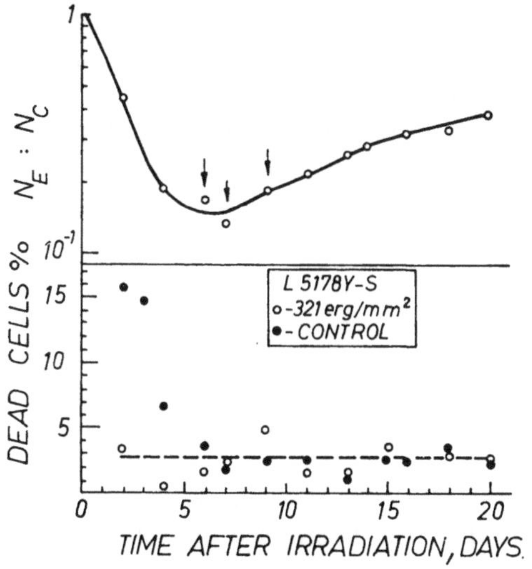

Fig. 1. Post-UV-exposure disturbances of growth and viability, and estimation of survival by the modified method of ALEXANDER and MIKULSKI (1960). In the upper block: relative cell number, i.e. ratio of the number of cells in the exposed culture (N_E) to the number of cells in the control culture (N_C) as a function of time. UV-light induced stimulation occured in the period following 6th day after the exposure. In the bottom block: viability changes. Arrows indicate relative cell number values used for estimation of survival.

When viability reached the control level, first two or three values of the relative cell number were taken as a basis of the survival estimation.
In the case of L5178Y-S cells, survival was additionaly determined by cloning in agar supplemented medium according to GILBERT and FOX (1966) with own modifications (BEER and SZUMIEL 1975). In split-dose experiments, appropriate corrections based on direct counts were made to allow for growth of the cell populations between the exposures. Our attempts to clone L5178Y-R cells have as yet been unsuccessful.

2.5. *Determination of ³H-TdR incorporation*

Cultures of 2×10^5 cells/ml were incubated for 0.5 h in the presence of [methyl-^{3}H] thymidine (2 μCi/ml, spec. activity 8 or 15.3 Ci/mmole, UVVVR, Praha, Czechoslovakia). Extraction of nuclear material was done by the method of BOSSMAN and BERNACKI (1970) with a following alteration: acid insoluble fraction after washing with ethanol: ethyl ether 2:1 was dried; dry precipitate was dissolved in 0.4 ml of trypsin solution (6 μg/ml of tris buffer pH 8.12) at 37 °C, under stirring. Radioactivity of so prepared samples was measured with an Intertechnique, France, liquid scintillation Counter, type SL-30. The results were related to the protein content determined according to LOWRY, ROSENBROUGH, FARR and RANDALL (1951).

2.6. *Labeling index determination*

The cultures were incubated for 1 h in the medium containing 2.5 μCi/ml of [methyl-^{3}H] thymidine (spec. activity 8 or 15.3 Ci/mmole, UVVVR, Praha, Czechoslovakia), washed with physiological saline and hypotonized with 0.075 M KCl for 15 min at room temperature. Hypotonized cells were fixed with acetic acid — ethanol (1:3 v/v) and spread on the microscopic slides. The slides were covered with Kodak stripping film (type AR 10) and exposed for 11 days at 4 °C. The developed slides were stained with 10% GIEMSA-solution. Three thousand cells were scored for determinatio of the labeling index.

3. Results

3.1. *UV-light sensitivity of L5178Y-R and L5178Y-S cells*

The cells of both strains were exposed to UV-light either in the FISCHER-medium or in the HANKS-solution and then their survival was determined by cloning or on the basis of growth and viability observations. Results of these determinations are presented in Fig. 2.
It can be seen that L5178Y-R cells are markedly more sensitive to UV-light than L5178Y-S cells. The initial shoulder occurs only on the survival curves for L5178Y-S cells.
These results confirm earlier observations (BEER, WALICKA 1971, BEER, SZUMIEL, WALICKA 1973 a, b).

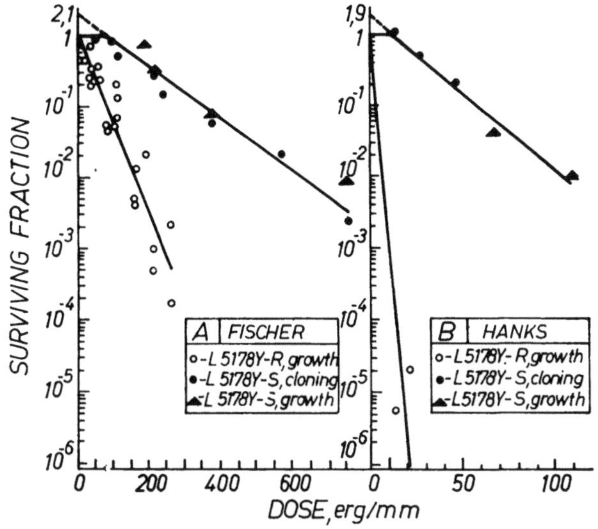

Fig. 2. Dose-survival relationships for L5178Y-R and L5178Y-S cell strains. Cells were irradiated in the FISCHER-medium (A), or in the HANKS-solution without phenol red (B). Method of survival determination indicated in the boxes. The curves, with exception of that for L5178Y-R cells irradiated in the HANKS-solution were calculated by the least square method. Mean lethal doses in the FISCHER-medium: 36 erg/mm² for L5178Y-R cells and 119 erg/mm² for L5178Y-S cells; in the HANKS-solution: ca. 2 erg/mm² for L5178Y-R cells and 20 erg/mm² for L5178Y-S cells.

3.2. *Split-dose effects*

The doses used in several series of split-dose experiments with L5178Y-R and L5178Y-S cells gave after the first UV-fraction survivals above 50% and after the cumulative doses ca. 20%. L5178Y-R cells were irradiated with 32 or 16 + 16 erg/mm². L5178Y-S cells were exposed to 214 or 107 + 107 erg/mm².

Relative survival, i.e. ratio of survivals after split-dose and cumulative-dose irradiations was determined. Results are presented in Fig. 3. It can be seen that fractionated irradiation caused in the two cell strains diametrically different changes of the relative survival.

In the case of L5178Y-S cells, intervals between the doses shorther than 7 h caused no change of the killing effect. Marked sparing effects were observed for longer intervals. A thirteen-hour interval was sufficient for complete recovery from sublethal damages caused by the first 107 erg/mm² fraction, as it can be concluded from the following calculation: for L5178Y-S cells expected survival after 107 erg/mm² is 66%; when all sublethal lesions are repaired in the interval between the doses, then after the second dose of 107 erg/mm² a survival of $0.66 \times 0.66 = 0.43 = 43\%$ is to be expected. Experimentally determined survivals were 78% for 13 h interval and 67% for 24 h interval. This indicates that after 13 h or longer interval the populations of L5178Y-S cells not only responded as the unexposed cells but in fact they seemed to be more UV-resistant.

Fractionation of UV-light caused in L5178Y-R cells a potentiation of the lethal effects with a minimum of the relative survival at a 4.5 h interval between the exposures.

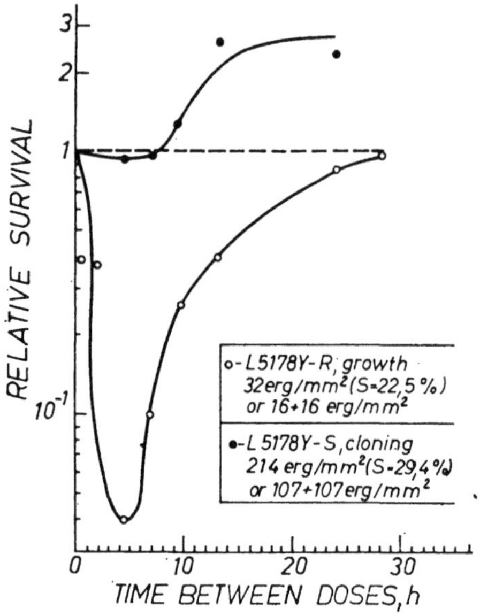

Fig. 3. Comparison of UV-light split dose effects on survival of L5178Y-R and L5178Y-S cells. In the boxes: S-survival after cumulative dose. Survivals after the first fraction estimated from dose-survival curves: 70% for L5178Y-R cells, 66% for L5178Y-S cells.

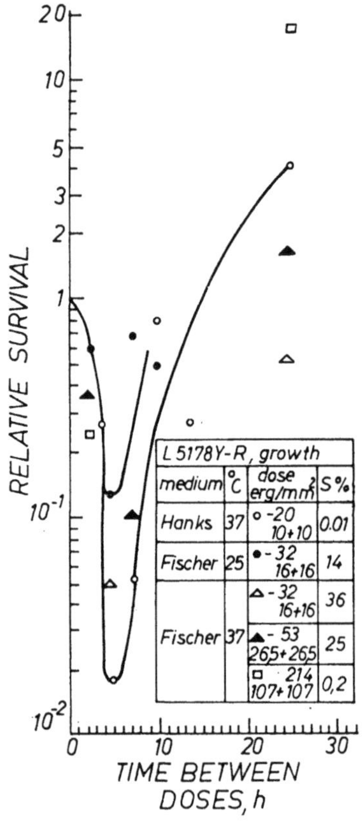

Fig. 4. Relative survival curves for L5178Y-R cells exposed to split-doses of UV-light under various conditions. HANKS: exposures of the cells in the HANKS-solution. 25 °C: incubation between the doses at 25 °C. S — survival after cumulative doses.

Lethal effects were smaller for longer intervals and relative survival reached values close to 1 for 24 h and 28 h intervals.
Potentiating effect of fractionation was observed for L5178Y-R cells exposed to UV-light under various conditions (Fig. 4): similar phenomena occured after lower and higher doses of UV-light, when the cells were irradiated in the HANKS-solution and when they were incubated between the exposures at 25°C. In this last case the potentiation was smaller than that observed for cells incubated at 37 °C.

3.3. UV-light induced growth disturbances

Growth disturbances induced by the first fraction of UV-light were observed in cultures of L5178Y-R cells exposed to 16 erg/mm² and in cultures of L5178Y-S cells exposed to 107 erg/mm². Results of these observations are summarized in Fig. 5. It can be seen

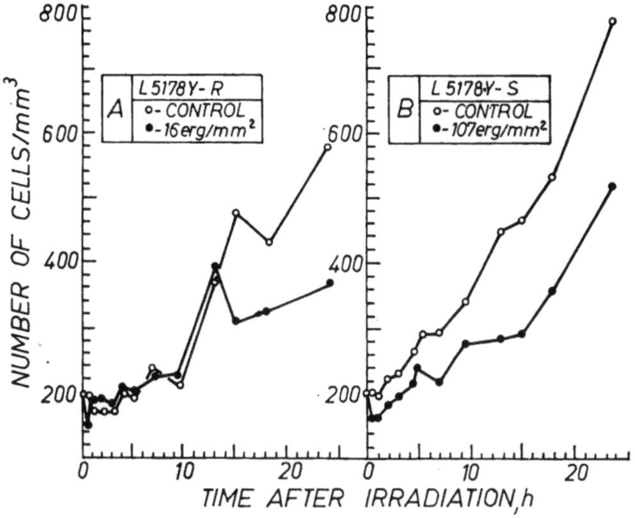

Fig. 5. UV-light-induced growth disturbances in L5178Y-R and L5178Y-S cell populations. The points represent mean values from three independent experiments.

that in all cultures, irradiated and non-irradiated, soon after beginning of the observation, a decrease in cell density was observed. This decrease is partly caused by handling (cf. RAUTH and WHITMORE 1966, SMITH and DENDY 1968, TODD, COOHILL, HELEWELL and MAHONEY 1969, TROSKO and CHU 1973). We found (unpublished observations) that L5178Y cell populations can partly lyse during centrifugation, transfer to fresh portions of medium, to buffered salt solutions, and upon change of temperature or pH. However, the decrease of cell density during first 30 min of the observations was markedly higher in the irradiated cultures. Soon after this decrease, in the case of L5178Y-R cells an increase in cell density was observed. The nature of these early variations is not clear at present.
We shall restrict the following considerations of the growth disturbances to a period corresponding to approx. one doubling time, following the early cell density variations

(1h). No deviations from normal viability, as determined by nigrosine staining, were observed in this period.
L5178Y-R cells (Fig. 5A) in the period between 1st and 13th hour after the exposure grew at a rate very close to the control one.
L5178Y-S cell populations (Fig. 5B) grew between 1st and 5th hour after the exposure at the control rate. Then, between 5th and 15th hour the cell growth was considerably retarded.

3.4. *^{3}H-TdR incorporation and labeling index*

^{3}H-TdR incorporation rate was determined at intervals after exposure to the first fraction of UV-light and compared with the control rate. Results of these determinations are presented in Fig. 6. It can be seen that 2 h after exposure ^{3}H-TdR incorporation

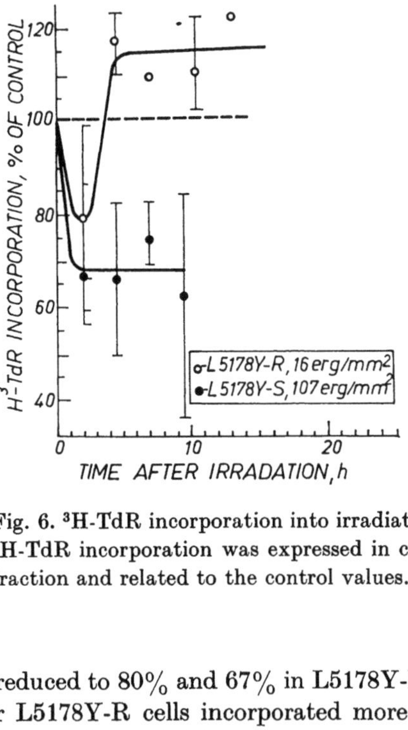

Fig. 6. ^{3}H-TdR incorporation into irradiated cultures of L5178Y-R and L5178Y-S cells. ^{3}H-TdR incorporation was expressed in counts/sec mg of protein in the acid insoluble fraction and related to the control values.

rate was reduced to 80% and 67% in L5178Y-R and L5178Y-S cells, respectively. Soon thereafter L5178Y-R cells incorporated more ^{3}H-TdR than the controls: on average 115% between 4.5 and 13th hour after the exposure. At the same time the incorporation rate into L5178Y-S cells remained at the reduced level: on average 67% between 2nd and 9th hour.
At 4.5 h after exposure labelling indices were determined of the irradiated and control cell populations. The results are presented in Table 2.
It can be seen that in both cell strains labeling indices were higher in the irradiated cell populations than in controls: on average by 9% in the case of L5178Y-R cells and by 18% in the case of L5178Y-S cells.

Table 2. Labeling indices (LI) at 4.5 h after irradiation. L5178Y-R cells irradiated with 16 erg/mm², L5178Y-S cells with 107 erg/mm².

Cell strain	Date of the experiment	LI of control, %	LI of irradiated population, %	Δ LI, %
L5178Y-R	20th Oct. 1973	53.8*	58.8**	+ 5.0
	11th Dec. 1973	36.0	46.6	+10.6
	14th Mar. 1974	36.4	46.5	+10.1
L5178Y-S	3rd Dec. 1974	49.0	69.1	+20.1
	10th Mar. 1974	65.0	81.3	+16.3

* 2,000 cells scored
** 1,250 cells scored

4. Discussion

4.1. *Differences in sensitivity to UV-light*

Since dosimetry of UV-light presents serious technical problems and mammalian cell cultures are irradiated in different laboratories under different conditions, the comparisons of data characterizing sensitivity to UV-light of various mammalian cells can be made only for the data obtained in the same laboratory. A selection of such data, including our own results is presented in Table 3. It can be seen that the difference between

Table 3. Differences in sensitivity to UV-light of some strains of mammalian cells cultivated in vitro.

Cell strains	Mean lethal dose (D_0), erg/mm²	Reference	Ratio of mean lethal doses
V79	43	CLEAVER, 1969	$D_0^{V79} : D_0^{V7979} = 1.43$
V7979	30		
Yoshida R	52	FOX, FOX 1973	$D_0^{\text{Yoshida R}} : D_0^{\text{Yoshida S}} = 4.00$
Yoshida S	13		
HeLa S3	87	ISOMURA, NIKAIDO, HORIKAWA, SUGAHARA, 1973	$D_0^{\text{HeLaS3}} : D_0^{\text{HeLaS3-S2M}} = 1.93$
HeLa S3-S4M	68		
HeLa S3-S2M	45		
HeLa S3	67	KLÍMEK, ŠEVČÍKOVÁ, VLASÍŇOVÁ, OLTOVÁ 1973	$D_0^{\text{HeLaS3-clone 18/2}} : D_0^{\text{HeLaS3-clone 46}} = 1.78$
HeLa S3-clone 18/2	80		
HeLa S3-clone 46	45		
Lich-M4	51	RANDTKE, WILLIAMS, LITTLE, 1972	$D_0^{\text{Lich-M4}} : D_0^{\text{Lich-10}} = 1.11$
Lich-10	46		
Normal fibroblasts (N)	22—29	CLEAVER, 1970	$D_0^{N} : D_0^{XP} = 2.44 \div 14.5$
XP fibroblasts (XP)	2—9	GOLDSTEIN, 1971	
L5178Y-S	119	This work	$D_0^{\text{L5178Y-S}} : D_0^{\text{L5178Y-R}} = 3.31$
L5178Y-R	36		

mean lethal doses for L5178Y-R and L5178Y-S cells is considerable in comparison with other groups of related cell strains: larger differences were reported only for Yoshida R and Yoshida S cells and for normal and xeroderma pigmentosum fibroblasts.

4.2. Recovery from sublethal damage and post-exposure disturbances

Available information does not enable a comprehensive interpretation of the results of fractionated irradiation of L5178Y-R and L5178Y-S cells with UV-light. It would be particularly important for such an interpretation to know how the differences in cell size affect the UV-light sensitivities and, especially, how UV-light sensitivities of both cell strains vary in their cell cycles. However, it should be mentioned that it does not seem likely that the very low survival observed for L5178Y-R cells after fractionated irradiation will find a plausible explanation on the basis of the cell cycle variations. On the whole, differences in radiation sensitivities of mammalian cells in different cell cycle phases are much smaller than those observed by us, reaching a 25 times factor in extreme cases.

Nevertheless the data on growth, ^{3}H-TdR incorporation and labeling index disturbances indicate some factors affecting sensitivity of the L5178Y cells to UV-light.

In the case of L5178Y-R cells, maximal sensitivity to UV-light coincided with growth inhibition and it was observed at the time when ^{3}H-TdR incorporation rate and labelling index were enhanced. These observations indicate occurence of complex cell cycle disturbances, possibly including stimulation of cell progression through one or more stages of the cell cycle. Stimulating effects of UV-light on mammalian cells have been observed in various mammalian cell systems: promotion of $G1 \rightarrow S$-phase transition was reported for human kidney T cells by Bootsma and Humphrey (1968); Waldren and Johnson (1974) by exposure to UV-light induced to $G1$ chromatin of HeLa cells changes characteristic to S-phase; Walicka and Beer (1973) described for L5178Y cells growth stimulating effects of UV-light. Further studies will be needed for elucidation of the mechanisms underlying these phenomena.

It is interesting to compare results of the split-dose experiments with the data on the post-exposure incorporation of ^{3}H-TdR (Figs. 3, 4 and 6): although early increase of UV-light sensitivity was accompanied by a decrease in the DNA synthesis rate, later potentaiting effect, including its maximum, occured while ^{3}H-TdR was incorporated at a rate somewhat higher than the normal one.

Similar, although quantitatively less pronounced potentiation of lethal effects caused by UV-dose fractionation was reported for M3-1 cells by Todd, Coohill, Helewell and Mahoney (1969) and for V79-4 cells by Thilly and Heidelberger (1973). The latter authors noticed that increased lethality was accompanied by an increase in frequency of mutations towards 8-azaguanine resistance.

Disturbances of ^{3}H-TdR incorporation into L5178Y-R cells have an atypical character. For many strains of mammalian cells it was observed that DNA synthesis is strongly inhibited for several hours after exposure to UV-light and it was concluded that ^{3}H-TdR uptake measurement can serve as a more sensitive indicator of UV-effects than the colony forming ability assay in the low dose range (for review see Rauth 1970). In the case of L5178Y-S cells post-UV-exposure growth inhibition was accompanied by slown down incorporation of ^{3}H-TdR (2nd to 9th hour after the exposure, Fig. 6). These observations together with the increase of labeling index at 4.5 h indicate inhibition of DNA synthesis and a slown down progression of the cells through the *S*-phase. It is worth noticing that the sparing effect was observed for times when both growth and ^{3}H-TdR incorporation were inhibited.

Combined observations for L5178Y-R and L5178Y-S cells comply with the observations of HUMPHREY, SEDITA and MEYN (1970), and HUMPHREY and MEYN (1972), DOMON and RAUTH (1973) and TODD (1973) that the recovery from UV-sublethal damage is *S*-phase dependent. Additionally, our observations seem to indicate that retardation of traverse, through this phase of the cell cycle presents an important factor promoting the recovery from sublethal damages induced by UV-light.

This work was performed within the framework of the CMEA — Research Programme in Biophysics, Problem No. V.

Summary

Murine leukaemic lymphoblasts L5178Y-R and L5178Y-S were exposed to cumulative and split doses of 254 nm UV-light. Sensitivity to UV-light of the two strains varies markedly: mean lethal doses are 36 erg/mm^2 for L5178Y-R and 119 erg/mm^2 for L5178Y-S cells. This difference is accompanied by diametrically different effects of dose fractionation. In the case of L5178Y-S cells, for times between doses longer than 13 h, marked sparing effect was observed; whereas for L5178Y-R cells a considerable potentation of the lethal effects occured with a maximum at 4.5 h interval between exposures. Doses used in these experiments (214 or 107 + 107 erg/mm^2 for L5178Y-S cells and 32 or 16 + 16 erg/mm^2 for L5178Y-R cells) allowed to survive more than 50% of the cells after the first fraction and ca. 25% after the cumulative irradiation.

Disturbances were determined of growth, labelling index and tritiated thymidine (^{3}H-TdR) incorporation following the first doses used in the fractionation experiments. L5178Y-S cells incorporated less ^{3}H-TdR than control between the 2nd and 9th hour after exposure. Simultaneous increase of labelling index indicates slown down progression through the *S*-phase of the cell cycle. These disturbances coincided with the period of occcurance of the sparing effect. In the case of L5178Y-R cells maximal split dose potentating effect was observed when no growth inhibition occured, and ^{3}H-TdR incorporation rate and labelling index were enhanced. These data seem to indicate that retardation of traverse through *S*-phase of the cell cycle presents an important factor promoting the recovery from sublethal damages induced by UV-light.

A modified technique is described of survival determination by growth curve backward extrapolation. The modification takes into account viability changes.

References

[1] ALEXANDER, P., MIKULSKI, Z. B.: Biochem. Pharmacology **5**, 275 (1960)

[2] ALEXANDER, P., MIKULSKI, Z. B.: Nature **192**, 572 (1961)

[3] BEER, J. Z., BOCIAN, E., BUDZICKA, E., SZUMIEL, I., ZIEMBA-ŻAK, B., KOPEĆ, M.: Nukleonika **19**, 835 (1974)

[4] BEER, J. Z., LETT, J. T., ALEXANDER, P.: Nature **199**, 193 (1963)

[5] BEER. J. Z., SZUMIEL, I., 1975, Inst. Nucl. Res. (Warsaw) Rept. 1506/X/B/A.

[6] Beer, J. Z., Szumiel, I., Walicka, M.: Studia Biophysica (Berlin) **36/37**, 175 (1973a)
[7] Beer, J. Z., Szumiel, I., Walicka, M.: Bull. Acad. Polon, Sci., Ser. Sci. Biol. **21**, 837 (1973b)
[8] Beer, J. Z., Walicka, M.: Nukleonika **16**, 573 (1971)
[9] Bossman, H. B., Bernacki, R. J.: Exptl. Cell Res. **61**, 379 (1970)
[10] Bootsma, D., Humphrey, R. M.: Mutation Res. **5**, 289 (1968)
[11] Cleaver, J. E.: Int. J. Radiat. Biol., **16**, 277 (1969)
[12] Cleaver, J. E.: Int. J. Radiat. Biol., **18**, 554 (1970)
[13] Courtenay, V. D.: Radiat. Res. **38**, 186 (1969)
[14] Domon, M., Rauth, A. M.: Radiat. Res. **55**, 85 (1973)
[15] Fischer, G. A.: Proc. Am. Assoc. Cancer Res. **2**, 201 (1957)
[16] Fischer, G. A., Sartorelli, A. C.: Meth. Med. Res. **10**, 247 (1964)
[17] Fox, B. W., Fox, M.: Int. J. Radiat. Biol. **24**, 497 (1973a)
[18] Fox, M., Fox, B. W.: Int. J. Radiat. Biol. **23**, 359 (1973b)
[19] Gilbert, C. W., Fox, M.: Int. J. Radiat. Biol. **23**, 336 (1966)
[20] Goldstein, S.: Proc. Soc. Exp. Biol. Med. **37**, 730 (1971)
[21] Han, A., Miletić, B., Petrović, D.: Int. J. Radiat. Biol. **8**, 187 (1964)
[22] Humphrey, R. M., Meyn, R. E. 1972, in Molecular and Cellular Repair Processes, Fifth International Symposium on Molecular Biology, Baltimore, Maryland, June 3—4, 1971, The Johns Hopkins University Press, Baltimore, p. 159
[23] Humphrey, R. M., Sedita, B. A., Meyn, R. E.: Int. J. Radiat. Biol. **18**, 61 (1970)
[24] Isomura, K., Nikaido, O., Horikawa, M., Sugahara, T.: Radiat. Res. **53**, 143 (1973)
[25] Klímek, M., Ševčíková, P., Vlašínová, M., Oltová, A.: Studia Biophysica (Berlin) **36/37**, 149 (1973)
[26] Lett, J. T., Alexander, P.: Progr. Biochem. Pharmacol. **1**, 41 (1965)
[27] Lett, J. T., Parkins, G., Alexander, P., Ormerod, M. G.: Nature **203**, 593 (1964)
[28] Lowry, O. H., Rosenbrough, N. J., Farr, A. L., Randall, L. J.: J. Biol. Chem. **193**, 265 (1951)
[29] Paul, J., 1960, Cell and Tissue Culture, Edinburgh: E. and S. Livingstone Ltd.
[30] Randtke, A. S., Williams, J. R., Little, J. B.: Exptl. Cell Res. **70**, 360 (1972)
[31] Rauth, A. M.: Curr. Top. Radiat. Res. **4**, 195 (1970)
[32] Rauth, A. M., Whitmore, G. F.: Radiat. Res. **28**, 84 (1966)
[33] Shugar, D., 1966, in: The Nucleic Acids, Chargaff. E., Davidson, J. N. eds., vol. III, Academic Press, New York, p. 39
[34] Smith, C. L., Dendy, P. P.: Cell Tissue Kinet. **1**, 225 (1968)
[35] Thilly, W. G., Heidelberger, C.: Mutation Res. **17**, 287 (1973)
[36] Todd, P.: Radiat. Res. **55**, 93 (1973)
[37] Todd, P., Coohill, T., Helewell, A. B., Mahoney, J.: Radiat. Res. **38**, 321 (1969)
[38] Trosko, J. E., Chu, E. H. Y.: Chem. Biol. Interactions **6**, 317 (1973)
[39] Waldren, C. A., Johnson, R. T.: Proc. Natl. Acad. Sci. USA **71**, 1137 (1974)
[40] Walicka, M., 1975, Krzyżowa wrażliwość komórek L5178Y-R i L5178Y-S na promieniowanie X i światło UV (Cross-sensitivity of L5178Y-R and L5178Y-S cells to X-rays and UV-light), Ph. D. Thesis Inst. Nucl. Res., Warszawa
[41] Walicka, M., Beer, J. Z.: Studia Biophysica (Berlin) **36/37**, 165 (1973)

DNA Repair in Barley after the Action of Methyl Nitrosourea and Sulphonic Acid Esters

J. Velemínský, V. Pokorný, T. Gichner, J. Šatava and J. Švachulová

Institute of Experimental Botany, Czechoslovak Academy of Sciences,
Praha 6, Flemingovo 2, Czechoslovakia

In embryos of barley seeds, DNA single-strand breaks were detected immediately after the treatment with MNU. No alkali-labile sites (apurinic sites) were detected in isolated DNA at this stage. The DNA single strand breaks are reparable by a prereplication type of repair, especially when air storage of seeds with 30% water content, submerse seed storage or longer post-treatment seed washing were applied after MNU treatment and before the seed germination. This repair is connected with the recovery from MNU induced seedling height reduction and the rate of repair and recovery is dependent on the dose of MNU and duration of seed storage. The caffeine potentiation of EMS-induced biological injury was accompanied by a smaller size of newly synthesized DNA single strands in comparison to the size of these DNA strands following EMS treatment alone. This probably indirectly demonstrates a second type of repair, acting during or after the DNA synthesis.

1. Introduction

Although not yet fully understood, the reaction between induced mutagenesis and carcinogenesis by chemical is commonly accepted. Especially the initiation steps, i.e. the induction of lesions in DNA, their recognition by repair enzymes and subsequent error free or error prone repair seems to play an important role in both processes (cf. Trosko and Chu 1975). In spite of great differences between prokaryotic organisms, eukaryotic microorganisms and other organisms including mammalian cells, the mechanism of in vivo interaction of chemical mutagens and carcinogens with DNA and the consequent repair of induced lesions differ only in minor details (cf. Howard-Flanders 1973). In this report we will try to demonstrate that these interactions and repairs are similar in higher plants.

Carcinogenic alkyl nitrosoureas and sulphonic acid esters are very potent mutagens in higher plants. In barley they induce recessive gene mutations, chromosome aberrations, sterility of spikes, reduction of seedling growth and — at higher concentrations — depression of seed germination (Gichner and Gaul 1971, Gichner et al. 1971). All these effects are correlated with each other, dependent on dose of the mutagen and — at suitable conditions — reparable. This reparability (recovery) is especially strong, when special conditions are applied after the mutagenic treatment of seeds before the onset of germination. All these conditions favouring recovery, either prolong the period between the mutagenic treatment and *S*-phase or remove the residual, not yet reacting mutagen from seeds, or both. We have already published elsewhere that this recovery, strengthened by the mentioned posttreatment conditions, was connected with the repair of DNA single-strand breaks (SSB) and/or alkali labile sites induced by mutagen in embryonic cells (Velemínský et al., 1972, 1973, Zadražil et al. 1974).

On the other hand the changes in the amount of DNA 7-methyl-guanine seem not to be connected with the repair (VELEMÍNSKÝ et al. 1973).
The method by which the DNA repair was followed, i.e. the sedimentation in alkaline sucrose gradients, cannot distinguish, whether single-strand breaks or alkali labile sites or both are repaired in vivo. The reason for this failure is that alkaline conditions of gradients convert alkali labile sites to SSB in vitro. In this communication we present results distinguishing the role of both lesions. Furthermore we will characterize this type of DNA repair especially with respect to its dependence on dose of the mutagen and duration of repair-favouring conditions. Last but not least indirect evidence bearing on the existence of another type of repair in barley (most probably of the postreplication type) is presented.

2. Material and methods

Chemicals. Abbreviation use: EMS — ethyl methanesulphonate, [^{3}H]TdR — thymidine ^{3}H (spec. act. 19.4 Ci/mmole), MMS — methyl methanesulphonate, MNU — N-methyl-N-nitrosourea, SSC — standard saline citrate (0.15M NaCl, 0.015M sodium citrate).
Scheme of treatment and repair favouring conditions: is given in Fig. 1.

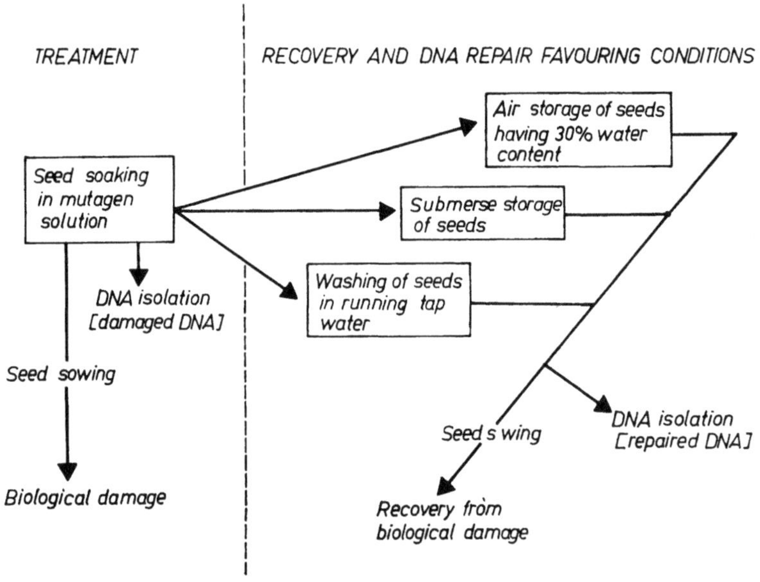

Fig. 1

All procedures were carried out at 25 °C, except for seed drying to 30% water content (40 °C). Constant water content of seeds during the air-storage was kept by seed storage above water in closed vessels. Submerse storage was enabled by keeping the seeds under distilled water bubbled with nitrogen. During these posttreatment conditions the seeds did not germinate although during air storage comparatively high enzyme activity in seeds was observed (ŠVACHULOVÁ et al. 1975). The degree of biological damage was expressed by the seedling height reduction (cf. GICHNER et al. 1971).

DNA was isolated after the mutagenic treatment or after the end of repair favouring conditions from seed embryos by modified Marmur's method (VELEMÍNSKÝ et al. 1973). The control DNA was isolated from water presoaked barley seed embryos. Detection of SSB and/or alkali labile sites was carried out by sedimentation analysis of DNA (dissolved in SSC) in alkaline sucrose gradients (5—20% sucrose w/v in 0.9M NaCl, 1 mM EDTA, 0.3M NaOH). After centrifugation at 5 °C in Spinco L2-65B, rotor SW 27.1 or SW 56 Ti, the gradients were removed from the top by Buchler Auto Densi-Flow and measured and recorded in a differential UV analyzer.
Distinction between SSB and alkali labile sites: According to Ts'o et al. (1962) formamide denatured DNA without inducing strand breakage. GAUDIN and YIELDING (1972) proposed to use formamide gradients to distinguish alkali-labile sites in alkylated DNA. To enable the simplier absorbancy measurement of DNA we have used neutral gradient of 1—15% (w/v) sucrose dissolved in 80% formamide (with 1 M Tris-HCl buffer pH 7.4). The centrifugation was carried out in SW 56 Ti rotor (gradient length 5.5 cm) at 55000 rev./min for 6 hours at 25 °C. DNA, layered on the gradient was dissolved in 80% formamide pH 7.4. A lower sedimentation rate of DNA in this gradient indicates the occurrence of SSB. To detect the relative amount of alkali-labile sites, DNA samples dissolved in 80% formamide were mixed with 1 N NaOH (3 : 1 v/v), incubated at 37° 30 min, neutralized with 1 N HCl. The alkali labile sites should be thus converted to SSB (cf. STRAUSS et al. 1968). The sedimentation pattern of this DNA in formamide-sucrose gradient was then compared with the sedimentation pattern of the same DNA sample, preincubated in neutral conditions (dist. H_2O instead of NaOH). Lower sedimentation rate of DNA, preincubated with NaOH indicates the presence of alkali labile sites, provided the difference is higher than in similarly preincubated samples of intact (control) DNA. An experiment with calf thymus DNA yield the following results: Difference between the peak center of sedimentation curves of DNA, preincubated with NaOH and without it involved 0.5 mm, the same difference of similarly preincubated apurinic DNA (50 mM MMS 30 min depurinated at 50° 6 h) involved 10 mm.
Sedimentation analysis of newly synthesized DNA: Mutagen treated or control seeds were allowed to germinate in Petri dishes with blotted paper saturated with [^{3}H]TdR (5 μCi/ml), for 3 days. DNA isolated as usually was centrifugated in alkaline sucrose gradient, SW 27.1 rotor of Spinco L2-65B, 20 drop fraction were collected, mixed with toluene: Triton X-100 (2:1), 4 g PPO, 0.1 g POPOP per liter) and radioactivity, characterizing the newly synthesized DNA, was measured with scintillation counter Mark I.

3. Results and discussion

I. Sedimentation studies on preformed DNA

DNA isolated form barley seed embryos after the mutagenic treatment, either before or after repair favouring conditions, represents the old DNA preformed before the mutagenic treatment. This assumption is supported by our observation that there is negligible incorporation of [^{3}H]TdR into nuclei of MNU-treated barley embryonic cells during the air-storage (unpubl.), very low incorporation into DNA at the end of 24 h washing (FOUSOVÁ et al. 1974). Moreover, air-stored or submerse stored seeds apparently do not germinate and DNA synthesis starts first after the apparent onset of germination (VELEMÍNSKÝ et al. 1973).

Treatment of seeds with MNU and three subsequent conditions (air- or submerse storage, washing) influence the sedimentation pattern of this preformed DNA in alkaline sucrose gradients. Lower sedimentation rate of DNA in MNU treated seeds (Fig. 2a, b, c, curve 1) indicates the induction of single-strand breaks and/or alkali-labile sites. Higher sedimentation rate of DNA in MNU treated and air stored (Fig. 2a), washed (b) and submerse-stored (c, curve 2) seeds indicates the repair of these lesions during the post-treatment conditions.

As previously stated the alkaline sucrose gradient method cannot distinguish if the repaired lesions are single strand breaks, alkali labile sites or both. Identification of the repaired lesion is possible at neutral DNA denaturation i.e. with neutral sucrose-formamide gradient. Sedimentation curves of DNA presented in Fig. 2c and d demonstrated similar sedimentation pattern in alkaline sucrose and in neutral sucrose-formamide gradients. Thus SSB were found in vivo immediately after the tretament with MNU

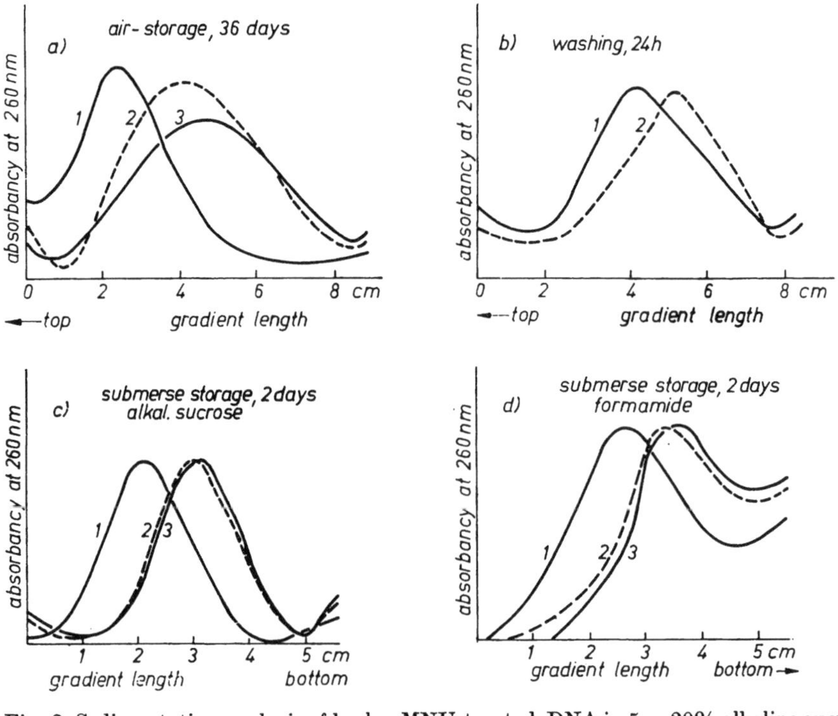

Fig. 2. Sedimentation analysis of barley MNU-treated DNA in 5 — 20% alkaline sucrose gradient. Curve 1 — DNA isolated after MNU treatment. Curve 2 — DNA isolated after MNU treatment and repair favouring-conditions. Curve 3 — control barley DNA.

a. seed treatment: 10 h water soaking, 3 h 8 mM MNU, air-storage 35 days. Centrifugation Spinco rotor SW 27.1 25000 rev./min 19 h 5 °C.

b. treatment: 4 mM MNU 5 h, 19 h washing. Centrifugation MSE superspeed centrifuge, 6×16 ml rotor, 23000 rev./min 18 h 6 °C.

c. treatment: 7.5 mM MNU 5 h 2 days submerse storage under water bubbled with N_2. Centrifugation Spinco rotor SW 56 Ti, 55000 rev./min 5 °C 3 h.

d. treatment as given under c., centrifugation Spinco rotor SW 56 Ti 55000 rev./min, 25 °C 6 h.

(5—6 hours) and are repaired during 2 days of storage. Similar results were obtained in all other experiments with submerse and air storage.
It is well known that with in vivo alkylated DNA, alkali labile apurinic sites are formed from alkylated DNA bases, and SSB arise from apurinic sites-both either spontaneously or through action of specific endonucleases (cf. CERUTTI 1974, LAWLEY 1974).
At least two endonucleases have been isolated in bacteria and mammalian cells which can recognize apurinic sites, one of which is able to also recognize some alkylated bases in DNA (VERLY et al. 1973, LJUNGQUIST and LINDAHL 1974, KIRTIKAR and GOLDTHWAIT 1974). As the half life of spontaneous backbone breakage at apurinic sites is rather long (cf. LAWLEY 1966) the occurrence of SSB just after the treatment must be ascribed preferentially to the action of one or both specific endonucleases mentioned. In Phaseolus such an endonuclease was claimed to be found (VERLY et al. 1973). The isolation of a similar endonuclease in barley is now underway in our laboratory.
Which part of alkali-labile sites remains unchanged to single-strand breaks in the period of treatment or during the repair process? This was elucidated by comparing the sedimentation pattern in sucrose-formamide gradient of NaOH (alkali)-preincubated and water (neutral)-preincubated DNAs. The results are summarized in Table 1. In DNA isolated from MNU treated and unstored seeds the difference between peak centres of neutral and alkali-preincubated samples was as negligible as in the control (intact) DNA. In DNA isolated from MNU treated and submerse stored seeds this difference

Table 1. Distinction of DNA alkali-labile sites from single-strand breaks by sedimentation in 80% formamide with neutral sucrose gradient.

Exp.	Treatment with MNU	Storage days	DNA peak centre (mm, from the top) in gradients			Difference 2—3
			5—20% alkal. sucrose	80% formamide with 1—15% sucrose		
				neutral preincubation	alkaline preincubation	
I.	7.5 mM, 5 h	0	16.3	28.8	28.3	0.5
	7.5 mM 5 h	2 (subm.)	20.3	31.6	29.3	2.3
	H_2O	0	22.3	32.1	31.4	0.7
II.	10 h H_2O, 6 mM, 3 h	0	27.5	20.3	19.8	0.5
	10 h H_2O, 6 mM, 3 h	28 (air)	36.3	22.8	21.4	1.4
	H_2O	0	47.7	24.4	24.1	0.3

Alkaline preincubation of DNA before layering on formamide gradients — exp. I: 3 vol. of DNA, dissolved in 80% formamide, mixed with 1 vol. 1N NaOH, incubated 30 min at 37 °C, neutralized with 1 vol. 1 N HCl. Exp. II: 2 vol. of DNA in SSC mixed with 1 vol. 1 N NaOH, incubated 15 min 37 °C. Neutral preincubation: instead of NaOH and HCl dest. H_2O was used — otherwise as in alkaline preincubation. Centrifugation: Spinco L2-65B, rotor SW 56 Ti (gradient length 5.5 cm) 55000 rev./min. Formamide gradients — exp. I; 25 °C, 6 h; exp. II: 25 °C, 4 1/2 h. Alk. sucrose gradients — exp. I: 5 °C 3 h; exp. II: rotor SW 27.1 (gradient length 9.5 cm) 25000 rev./min, 5 °C 19 h.

slightly increased. We thus can suppose that most if not all apurinic sites in vivo are transformed to SSB. Similar results were obtained in MNU treated and air-stored seeds. The increase of alkali labile sites during the storage can be explained by further alkylation of DNA (and subsequent depurination) in the seeds caused by MNU which remained in seed tissue.

Therefore we can conclude that SSB are repaired only or preferentially in the course of air- or submerse storage. The rate of this repair is strongly dependent on the dose of mutagen and duration of repair favouring conditions. This is demonstrated in Fig. 3. The points in the dashed lines represent the distance of sedimentation curve centres (in alkaline sucrose gradients) of control DNA and DNA isolated from MNU-treated and air stored seeds. In full lines the recovery from biological damage, measured by seedling

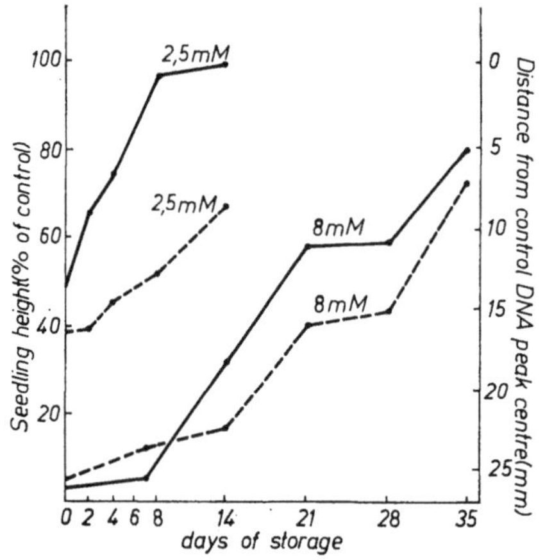

Fig. 3. Dose-dependence of DNA repair (dashed lines) and recovery from seedling height reduction (full lines). Treatment with MNU — 5 h, centrifugation in alkaline sucrose gradient (5—20%), Spinco rotor SW 27.1, 25000 rev./min 19 h 5 °C.

height, is expressed. With the increasing duration of storage, the sedimentation rate of DNA, as well as seedling height, approach the undamaged control. At the same concentration of MNU the slope of recovery- and repair lines are parallel, at different MNU doses these lines possess different slopes. From the given values the rate of repair and recovery can be calculated as a percentage of damage recovered or repaired per day of storage. As 100% we take the degree of damage found in MNU treated, unstored seeds. The values found in untreated seeds represent zero percent. After 2.5 mM MNU (3 h on 10 h presoaked seeds) 6.4% of seedling height was recovered and 5.9% of SSB was repaired per day of seed storage. In 8 mM MNU treated seeds (3 h, on 10 h water presoaked seeds) these values are 2.2% of recovery and 2.1% of repair per day.

II. Repair in newly synthesized DNA

The foregoing data present evidence favouring the existence of DNA repair in performed and damaged DNA. In bacteria and mammalian cells other repair system also occurs, called either recombination or postreplication repair, which is able to repair gaps in daughter DNA strands, synthesized on damaged templates (cf. HOWARD-FLANDERS 1974, LEHMANN 1974). The consequence of these gaps is a lower sedimentation rate of newly synthesized DNA in alkaline sucrose gradients; the consequence of postreplication repair is the increase of this size. A prerequisite of direct proof of postreplication repair is among others the possibility of synchronizing the cell cycle, which is not possible in cells of barley embryo. Nevertheless it seems probable that we can demonstrate the presence of similar repair indirectly in experiments with caffeine as a posttreatment agent.

In higher plants caffeine potentiates the action of ionizing radiation as well as of alkylating agents. This is expressed by enhancement of the frequency of chromosome aberrations (cf. KIHLMAN et al. 1974), seedling height reduction (AHNSTRÖM 1974, GICHNER and VELEMÍNSKÝ 1974) etc. Although it was assumed that this potentiation is caused by the inhibition of DNA repair (cf. KIHLMAN 1974), the molecular evidence was lacking in plants. We have therefore performed the following experiment: After the treatment of nongerminating barley seeds with EMS, caffeine in nontoxic dose was applied and the size of old DNA (isolated from nongerminating seeds) as well as of newly synthesizedDNA (isolated from germinating seeds) was followed (cf. VELEMÍNSKÝ et al. 1975). The main results are summarized in Table 2.

Table 2. Effect of caffeine posttreatment on the size of preformed and newly synthesized DNA.

Treatment	Seedling height (% of control)	Centre of DNA peak in ASG (mm from control)	
		preformed DNA	newly synth. DNA
EMS + H_2O	76	10.7	2.5
EMS + caffeine	5	11.5	10.3
H_2O + caffeine	98	2.7	0.7
H_2O + H_2O	100	0	0

Treatment conditions: 140 mM EMS 5 h, 18 h washing, 10 mM caffeine 3 h.
Centrifugation: 5—20% alkaline sucrose gradient (ASG) (pH 12.9).
Spinco L2-65B, rotor SW 27.1 (gradient length 9.5 cm) at 24000 rev./min, 5°C, 19 h.

The reduction of seedling height, induced by EMS, was strongly increased by caffeine posttreatment. The size of old DNA in alkaline sucrose gradient was not, however, influenced by caffeine posttreatment. Both DNA from EMS treatment and DNA from EMS and caffeine treatment sedimented more slowly than the control old DNA. In contrast, the newly synthesized, [^{3}H]TdR labelled DNA from EMS treated seeds sedimented in a pattern similar to the newly synthesized control DNA. The difference between the sedimentation pattern of control DNA and newly synthesized DNA from EMS + caffeine treatment remained, however as high as in the case of the old DNA. In accordance with similar results observed in mammalian cells (LEHMANN and KIRK-BELL 1974) we assume that as in mammalian cells, caffeine inhibits or delays a repair system which acts either during or after DNA synthesis in barley cells.

References

[1] Ahnström, G.: Mutation Res. **26**, 99 (1974)

[2] Cerutti, P. A.: Life Sci. **15**, 1567 (1974)

[3] Fousová, S., Velemínský, J., Gichner, T., Pokorný, V.: Biologia Plantarum (Praha) **16**, 168 (1974)

[4] Gaudin, D., Yielding, K. L.: Biochem. biophys. Res. Commun. **47**, 1396 (1972)

[5] Gichner, T., Gaul, H.: Radiation Botany **11**, 53 (1971)

[6] Gichner, T., Velemínský, J.: Mutation Res. **25**, 305 (1974)

[7] Gichner, T., Velemínský, J., Pokorný, V.: Mutation Res. **12**, 391 (1971)

[8] Howard-Flanders, P.: British med. Bull. **29**, 226 (1973)

[9] Kihlman, B. A.: Mutation Res. **26**, 53 (1974)

[10] Kihlman, B. A., Sturelid, S., Hartley-Asp, B., Nilsson, K.: Mutation Res. **26**, 105 (1974)

[11] Kirtikar, D. M., Goldthwait, D. A.: Proc. natn. Acad. Sci. U.S.A. **71**, 2022 (1974)

[12] Lawley, P. D.,: Prog. Nucl. Acid. Res. Mol. Biol. **5**, 89 (1966)

[13] Lawley, P. D.: Mutation Res. **23**, 283 (1974)

[14] Lehmann, A. R., Kirk-Bell, S.: Mutation Res. **26**, 73 (1974)

[15] Ljungquist, S., Lindahl, T.: J. biol. Chem. **249**, 1530 (1974)

[16] Strauss, B., Coyle, M., Robbins, S.: Cold Spring Harbor Symp. Quant. Biol., **33**, 277 (1968)

[17] Švachulová, J., Velemínský, J., Gichner, T.: Biologia Plantarum (Praha) **17**, 109 (1975)

[18] Trosko, J. E., Chu, E. H. Y.: Adv. in Cancer Res. **21**, 391 (1975)

[19] Ts'o, P. O., Helmkamp, G. K., Sander, C.: Biochem. biophys. Acta **55**, 584 (1962)

[20] Velemínský, J., Zadražil, S., Gichner, T.: Mutation Res. **14**, 259 (1972)

[21] Velemínský, J., Zadražil, S., Pokorný, V., Gichner, T., Švachulová, J.: Mutation Res., **17**, 49 (1973)

[22] Velemínský, J., Zadražil, S., Pokorný, V., Gichner, T., 1974, in: Polyploidy and induced mutations in plant breeding, IAEA, Vienna, 151.

[23] Velemínský, J., Gichner, T., Pokorný, V.: Mutation Res. 28, 79 (1975)

[24] Verly, W. G., Paquette, Y., Thibodeau, L.: Nature, New Biology **244**, 67 (1973)

[25] Zadražil, S., Pokorný, V., Velemínský, J., Gichner, T.: Biologia Plantarum (Praha) **16**, 7 (1974)

MODIFICATION OF DNA REPAIR BY EXOGENOUS FACTORS

Studies on Alterations of DNA Repair Processes

E. SCHRÖDER and E. MAGDON

Cancer Research Institute, Academy of Sciences of German Democratic Republic, Berlin-Buch

The repair of damaged DNA in normal and tumour cells is a fact that has been frequently demonstrated in the last decade.
Therefore, the search for possible influences on repair processes by exogenous factors that can considerably increase the sensitivity of a tumour cell by being specific repair inhibitors is a priority of current research work. These studies were based mainly on experimental-therapeutical considerations and were aimed at biological optimization of radiotherapy, in that certain substances administered in combination with the radiation treatment irreversibly inhibit the DNA repair in the tumours cells. A number of compounds from the literature and, to some degree, from our own experimental studies is listed:

(1) iodine compounds
(2) 2.4-dinitrophenol
(3) SH compounds
(4) hydroxyurea
(5) antirheumatics/detergents
(6) quinacrine/chloroquine
(7) bleomycin/actinomycin D
(8) caffeine

In addition the influence of hyperthermia on DNA repair was investigated.

Iodine compounds

The modification of biological radiation effects by iodine compounds has been described by several authors to consist in increasing the number of DNA lesions and adversely affecting their repair [47, 65, 66, 67, 68, 104]. The results listed in Table 1 were obtained essentially by investigating the repair of DNA single-strand breaks; only did VOICULETZ [104] study the influence of several iodine derivatives in the hydroxyurea-insensitive ^{3}H-thymidine incorporation in human lymphocytes.
Iodoacetate inhibits the repair only under oxic conditions, if it is present during the irradiation. It is assumed, therefore, that the substance effects a qualitative change of the radiation induced breaks, which inhibits the process of repair. In general, the sensibilization effect of iodine compounds is explained by an interaction of radiolytic products with the cell membrane which affects DNA synthesis and DNA repair.

Table 1. Effect of Iodine-compounds on DNA Repair.

Substance	Cells	Dose		Inhibition of Repair	Authors	
iodoacetate	*E. coli*			+	Noguti et al.	(1971)
	human fibroblasts	10^{-2} M		+	Kleijer et al.	(1973)
	human lymphocytes	10^{-2} M		+	Voiculetz et al.	(1975)
	E. coli	10^{-4} M		+	Nair et al.	(1976)
iodoacetamide	*E. coli*	2×10^{-3} M		+	Myers	(1971)
	E. coli	10^{-4} M		+	Myers et al.	(1973)
	human lymphocytes	10^{-5} M		+	Voiculetz et al.	(1975)
potassium iodide	*E. coli*	4×10^{-2} M		+	Myers	(1971)
	human lymphocytes	10^{-2} M		−	Voiculetz et al.	(1975)
potassium iodate	*B. subtilis*	3×10^{-4} M	a. irrad.	+	Noguti et. al.	(1971)
	B. subtilis	3×10^{-4} M	p. irrad.	−	Noguti et al.	(1971)
	E. coli	10^{-4} M		+	Myers et al.	(1973)
	human lymphocytes	10^{-3} M		−	Voiculetz et al.	(1975)

2.4-Dinitrophenol

Repair inhibition by 2.4-dinitrophenol (DNP) has been intensively investigated by Dalrymple et al. [13, 14, 63]. Using a concentration of 10^{-4} M he found complete inhibition of DNA repair following 10 krad in L-cells (Sanford's L-929 strain). Similar results were obtained by van der Schueren [86, 95] using a concentration of 3×10^{-3} M in *E. coli* irradiated with 20 krad, Kleijer [40] in T-cells and Ormerod [70] in L5178Y cells. In unirradiated cells DNP causes no alterations at the DNA (Fig. 1).

According to Palcic [88] and Dalrymple [14] the effect of DNP seems to depend on the medium being used, especially on the added serum, in the presence of which the substance is wholly ineffective. This finding may be responsible for the opposing results of Sawada and Okada [79] who worked with complete media. The repair inhibition by DNP is reversible, and undisturbed DNA repair starts immediately upon removal of the substance.

The negative influence of DNP on repair processes has to be related, in all probability, to the suppression of oxidative phosphorylation and, consequently, to the diminished supply of ATP in the cell. Owing to this disturbance of the cellular energy metabolism, ATP as a cofactor of the ligase reaction for joining the free ends in the damaged DNA is no longer available in sufficient quantity; hence, the process of repair can no longer be optimal [56]. On the other hand, additional supply of ATP is able to stimulate the repair process [53, 54, 105].

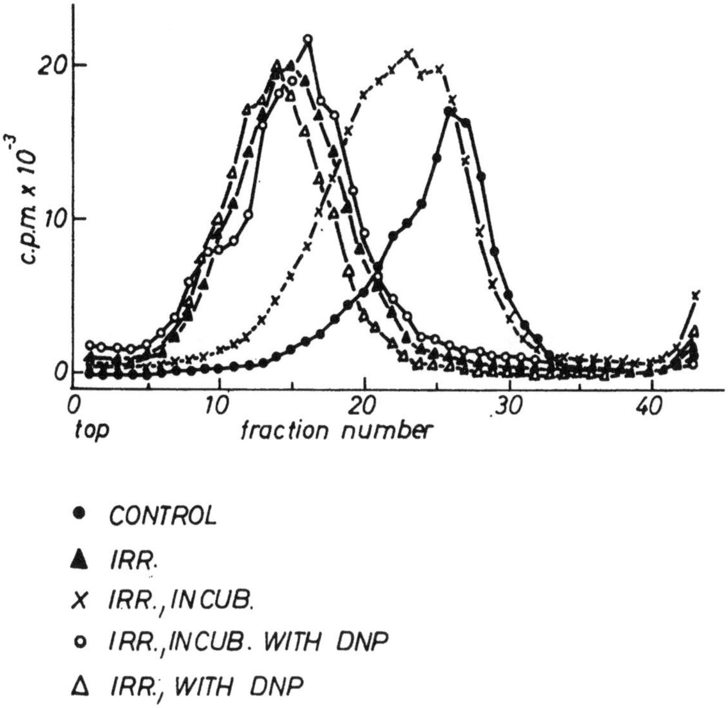

Fig. 1. Influence of DNP on the number of radiation-induced DNA breaks and the repair of single-strand breaks in T-cells (KLEIJER et al. 1973).

SH compounds

Low-molecular SH compounds are well-known mainly as radioprotectors, and have been intensively studied especially in the 50ies for their possible application in radiation therapy and in reactor accidents.

These substances have proved their radioprotective value in many biological systems both on molecular level and in totally irradiated animals. Efforts to elucidate their action mechanism have prompted a number of studies to investigate the interaction of these compounds with the cellular DNA but also with the alterations of DNA produced by irradiation. In particular, the effect of cysteamine (MEA) on the radiation-induced DNA break rate has been investigated on various objects. Thus, ROOTS [76] and SAWADA and OKADA [80] found a dose reduction factor (d.r.f.) of 6.0 for the number of radiation-induced DNA breaks, when mouse leukemia cells (L5178Y) were irradiated in the presence of MEA (50 mM).

A protection by MEA against radiation-induced DNA breaks was reported also by GINSBERG [25], LOHMAN et al. [49] on T-cells (32 mM MEA; d.r.f. 4.0) and *E. coli* K12 AB 1157 (44 mM MEA; d.r.f. 3.9) and VAN HEMMEN [30] on bacteriophage DNA (10 mM).

A factor of only 2.5 was obtained by PITRA et al. [71], irradiating Chinese hamster cells V79-4 in combination with MEA (50 mM). This comparatively low value is attributed by

these authors to the fact that the experiments were done not at 37° but at 0°. In contrast, Ormerod and Stevens [70] found at such low temperatures with L5178Y cells always the same number of DNA breaks irrespective of whether the irradiation was performed with or without MEA. MEA also affords protection against the induction of double-strand breaks both on bacteriophages [30, 81] and on mammalian cells (50 mM; d.r.f. 2.7) [71, 80].
Compared with other SH compounds MEA provides the best protection against DNA lesions; in contrast, when used in equimolar concentrations, l-cysteine, AET and cystamine are much less effective. But cystamine (50 mM) is also able to protect Chinese hamster cells against double-strand breaks [12]. Studies on the influence of these substances on DNA repair processes are fewer, and the results are in part contradictory. Sawada and Okada [80] found in mouse leukemia cells that cysteamine administered after irradiation with 10 krad affected the otherwise usual increase in molecular weight during afterincubation. In the concentration range between 5 and 500 mM the effective repair is reduced to about 60—30% of the irradiated but drug-free control. These findings could not be confirmed by Ormerod and Stevens [70] using the same cell strain, and in Chinese hamster cells too the rejoining of single-strand breaks was not inhibited [71].

Hydroxyurea

This compound has been repeatedly tested for its influence on processes of DNA repair so as to enable its application as an inhibitor of DNA synthesis in the investigation of unscheduled DNA synthesis.
Only did Kapp and Smith [32] find an irreversible inhibition of the increase in molecular weight during postirradiation incubation of *E. coli* K12 by impure samples of hydroxyurea (0.1 M), in contrast to untreated samples. But it can be taken for granted today that hydroxyurea in p.a. form (10^{-3}—10^{-2} M) does not affect the rejoining process of DNA strand breaks in irradiated cells [8, 79].
On the other hand, Fujiwara [18] found in L5 cells after UV-irradiation that postreplication repair was prevented by 2 mM hydroxyurea.

Antirheumatics/Detergents

The increasing contamination of the environment, but also the mounting uncontrollable ingestion of unrestricted drugs and long-lasting therapeutical procedures, e.g. with chronic early diseases, have prompted considerations to investigate the influence of pharmaceuticals on the intracellular repair system. This problem has been extensively dealt with by Altmann and his collaborators [16, 34, 35, 36, 37, 38, 39, 94, 101], studying in particular antirheumatic agents for their influence on DNA repair and semiconservative DNA synthesis.
The in vitro studies were carried out with lymphocytes of healthy donors and spleen cells of rat and mouse, and the hydroxyurea-resistant incorporation of ^{3}H-thymidine was measured after irradiation in the presence of the drug tested.
The substances under investigation were used in concentrations similar to the conventional therapeutical doses; overdoses were applied in a few cases only.

An experimental arrangement is illustrated in Figure 2. The results obtained with all substances tested are summarized in Table 2.
These findings were confirmed by the results of in vivo/in vitro studies, investigating lymphocytes from patients who were being treated for chronic polyarthritis for period of 7 months [16].
Table 3 shows that for D-penicillamine in both cases a strong inhibition of semiconservative DNA synthesis is obtained, whereas the DNA repair went completely unimpaired,

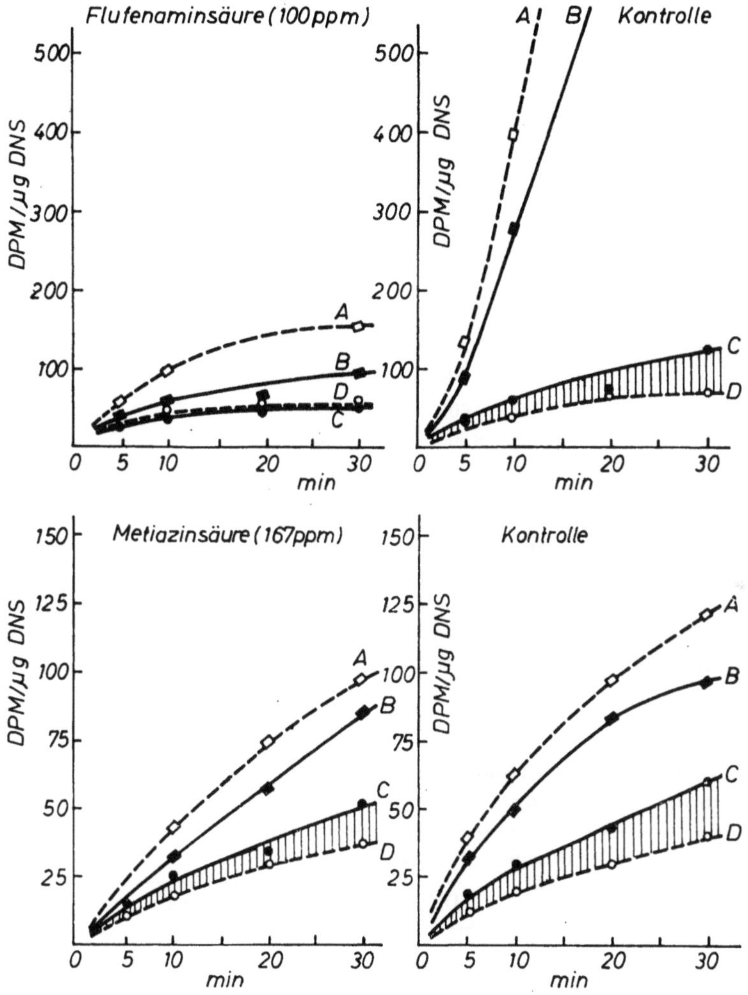

Fig. 2. Influence of flufenaminic- and metiazinic acid on the DNA synthesis and repair of spleen cells of mouse (KLEIN 1974).

A: DNA synthesis, control

B: DNA synthesis, irradiated

C: hydroxyurea, irradiated

D: hydroxyurea, control

Table 2. Influence of Antirheumatics on the DNA Synthesis and DNA Repair in Lymphocytes and Spleen Cells.

Substance	Dosage mg/d	Blood-level μg/ml	Inhibition of	
			DNA Synthesis	DNA Repair
D-penicillamin	750		++	—
metiazinic acid	1000	50	—	—
	3300	167	—	+
	5000	250	++	+++
kétoprofèn	200	11	—	—
	600	33	—	—
naproxen	375	50	—	+
	800	120	++	++
azapropazone	900	45	—	—
tolmetin	800	100	+	—
	1200	150	++	—
oxyphenbutazone	250	15	—	+
	600	50	+	++
flufenaminic acid	600	7	+	+
	8500	100	+++	+++
phenylbutazone		100	+++	+++
hydracillin		750	—	++
isonicotinic acid hydracide		100	++	—
procainamide		100	—	—

— no influence
\+ low inhibition
++ strong inhibition
+++ complete inhibition

Table 3. DNA Repair in Lymphocytes from Patients with Chronic Polyarthritis after Therapy.

Substance	Dosage mg/d	Inhibition of	
		DNA Synthesis	DNA Repair
azapropazone	900	—	—
prednisolon	7,5	++	++
D-penicillamin	750	++	—
indometacin	100	++	—
naproxen	500	—	+

— no influence
\+ low inhibition
++ strong inhibition

and naproxene exerted a very low action only on repair during the therapeutic treatment. The investigations have shown that most of the drugs tested here in doses common for clinical therapy have a low, if any, action in DNA repair.
Similar to drugs, the range of detergents being increasingly used in the pharmaceutical industry for the manufacture of various products, especially of cosmetics, has to be viewed as a permanent environmental factor so that possible remote effects resulting from diminished intracellular repair capacity cannot be ruled out. Hence, it was of interest to study the effects of these compounds on DNA metabolism. In human lymphocytes GAUDIN et al. [24] using Tween 80 (0.002%), Span 80 and Arlacel A (0.01%) found a 50% inhibition of UV-induced repair synthesis. Similar results were obtained by TUSCHL et al. [100] on ^{60}Co-irradiated mouse spleen cells with Tween 80, Nonidet P40 (octaphenolethyleneoxy-condensate) and Cremophor (reaction product of linseed oil with ethyleneoxide) and IVANOVA [64] on *Drosophila melanogaster*.
While Nonidet showed an effect already at a very low concentration of 0.005%, inhibition of unscheduled DNA synthesis was observable with Cremophor only from 0.015% onwards. Among the substances studied, Tween 80 is a specific repair inhibitor, while Nonidet and Cremophor inhibit both types of DNA synthesis to the same extent. In view of the wide-spread use of surface-active substances as emulsifiers of water insoluble pharmaceuticals it can be assumed that their co-carcinogenic effects are partly attributable to disturbed intracellular processes of recovery.

Quinacrine/Chloroquine

Quinacrine [2-methoxy-6-chloro-9(4-diethylamino-1-methylbuthyl)aminoacridine], which is used for therapy of malaria, belongs to the group of intercalating substances readily forming links with DNA. FUKS and SMITH [19] were the first to test the repairinhibiting action of the substance on bacteria (*E. coli* K-12 *rec*$^+$). In the presence of 0.15 mM quinacrine the repair of DNA single-strand breaks in irradiated bacterial cultures (20 krad) was suppressed completely and irreversibly, while the inhibition of post replication repair in UV-irradiated cells was reversible. Studies on mammalian cells led to similar results. In irradiated (30 krad) Chinese hamster cells (HA1) quinacrine (5 μg/ml) prevented recovery of damaged DNA, especially if the substance had been administered prior to treatment [103], as shown in Figure 3.
A total suppression of unscheduled DNA synthesis by quinacrine (4×10^{-5} M) was observed by VOICULETZ [104], MENEGHINI [59] and GAUDIN [23] in lymphocytes following γ- or UV-irradiation. The substance has no effects of its own unirradiated control cells but data reported on the modification of the break number are controversial. Unlike VOICULETZ [103], who found no increase in radiation-induced DNA breaks, REVESZ et al. [75] irradiating Chinese hamster cells in presence of quinacrine found an enhancement factor of 1.36.
The cytostatic action of chloroquine [7-chloro-4-(4-diethyl-amino-1-methylbuthyl-amino)chinoline], also a therapeutic agent in malaria therapy, in the combined treatment of solid animal tumours [21, 22] was also assumed to be in part due to inhibition of repair processes at the DNA. This hypothesis was confirmed by the studies of MICHAEL (61). The methylmethane sulfonate (MMS; 4 mM) induced DNA strand breaks of epithelial-like cells (ARL6) derived from a rat liver cell line were not mended in the pres-

ence of 0.2 mM chloroquine. At this concentration, chloroquine alone causes no lesion of the DNA. It is not known whether an interaction with the DNA or inhibition of protein synthesis is responsible for repair inhibition because much stronger blockers of protein synthesis, such as cycloheximide (0.018 mM), had no such potent action [59, 61, 77, 99] as shown in Figure 4.

It is not yet certain whether therapeutical doses of chloroquine, administered over longer periods of time, cause lesions to the cellular repair system. To be true, GAUDIN

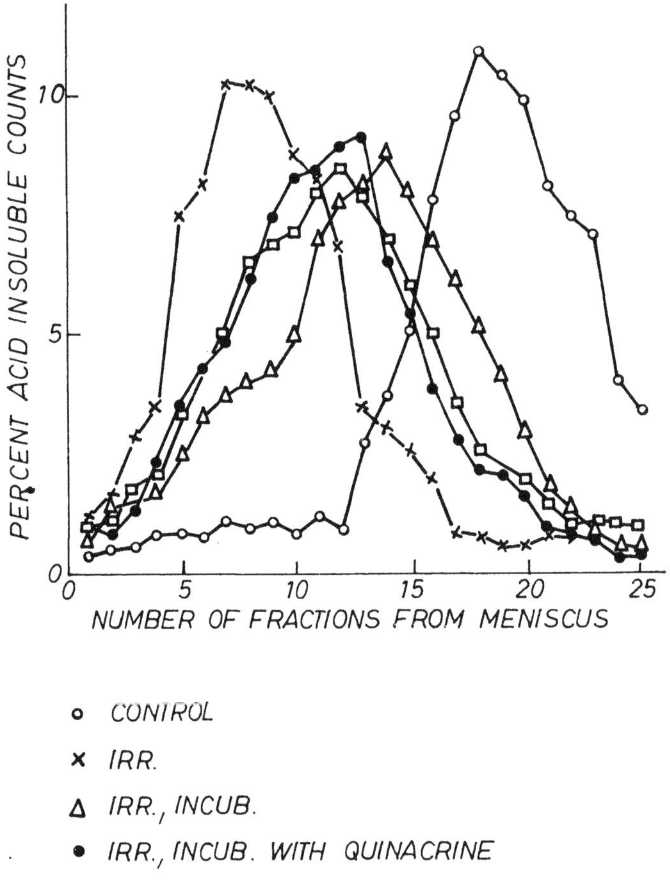

Fig. 3. Influence of quinacrine on the repair of DNA single-strand breaks (VOICULETZ 1974).

[23] observed in healthy human lymphocyte cultures and LOPEZ ZUMEL [50] on spleen cells after in vitro incubation with chloroquine (7×10^{-5} and 5×10^{-4} M, respectively) an about 50% inhibition of radiation-induced ^{3}H-thymidine incorporation, but HORKAY et al. [31] were unable to find any significant differences from pretherapeutical values in peripheral lymphocytes of patients with lupus erythematosus following a two-week's treatment with chloroquine (oral daily doses of 500 mg).

These findings are not consistent with the results obtained after in vitro incubation and are likely to be due to differences in the "real" concentration of the substance in the cell.

These studies suggest that the use of chinoline derivatives as sensitizers in tumour irradiation of man should be considered on account of their low toxicity and their selective accumulation in tumour tissues as established in animal experiments.

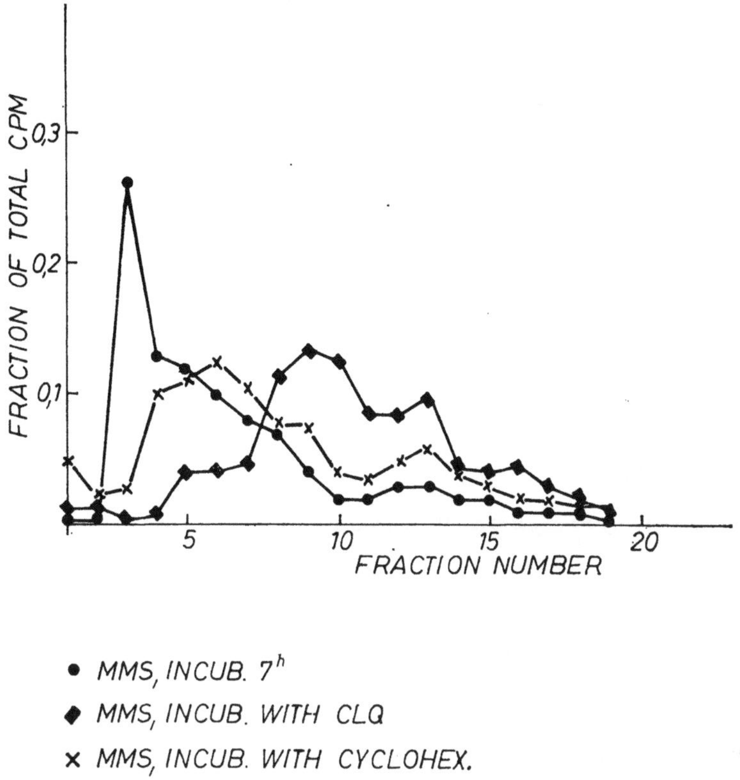

Fig. 4. Influence of chloroquine and cycloheximide on the repair of MMS-induced strand breaks (MICHAEL 1974).

Bleomycin/Actinomycin D

Bleomycin, an antibiotic which has been widely used for the therapy of malignant tumours since its discovery by UMEZAWA 1966, has also been studied for its influence on repair processes at the DNA [4, 6]. On account of its preferential accumulation in neoplastic cells, bleomycin could be appropriate to considerably improve the results of radiotherapy. It is difficult at present to give a realistic appraisal of the results obtained so far, because bleomycin itself causes single- and double-strand breaks at the DNA. Therefore, it has to be worked in such a concentration range in which the intrinsic effects of bleomycin do not yet appear (up to 0.5 μg/ml). BYFIELD et al. [6] found at this concentration in REQ cells only a low inhibition of break repair. Also, the repair replication in L1210 cells was inhibited by bleomycin (to 100 μg/ml) to a low extent only.
The DNA sedimentation profiles in Figure 5 show that the presence of bleomycin during afterincubation has only a low influence on the restitution of DNA; the highest deviation from the recovered specimen may have been masked already by a bleomycin-

induced effect. These investigations show that the hypothesis frequently put forward to explain the effect of bleomycin in case of combined treatment with X-rays plus bleomycin is not valid, and that similar DNA lesions as they are induced by irradiation are likely to be responsible for its effect.
Actinomycin D (Act. D), a specific inhibitor of RNA synthesis, is frequently used as a supporting agent in the polychemotherapy or as an adjuvant in radiotherapy for management of human noeplastic disease.

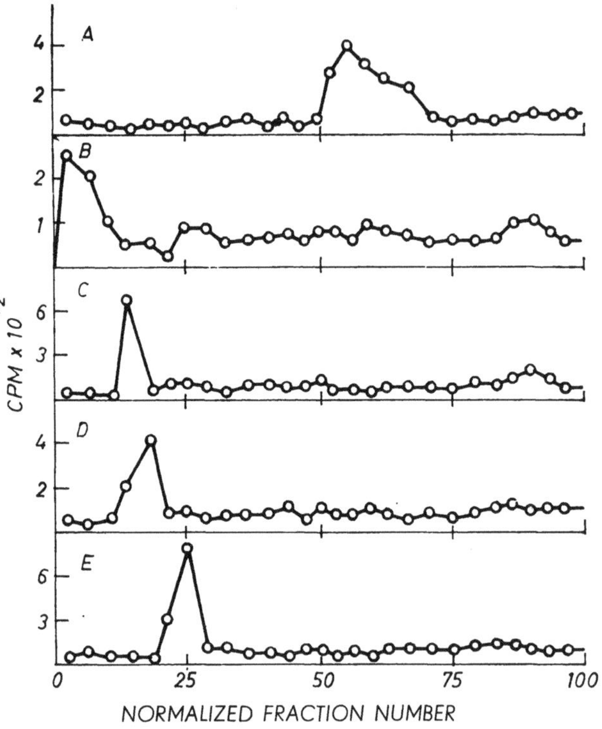

Fig. 5. Influence of bleomycin on the repair of DNA single-strand breaks (Byfield 1976).

A: irradiated, no incubation

B: irradiated, incubated for 60 min at 37°

C—E: irradiated, incubated for 60 min with 0.005, 0.1 and 0.5 μg bleomycin/ml

The combined action of Act. D and irradiation on cellular and molecular level has been studied in particular by Elkind [17], who was able to show that already a concentration of 0.002 μg/ml of this antibiotic applied in fractioned irradiation of cell cultures suppressed the repair of sublethal lesions.
The results on the action of Act. D on the repair of DNA strand breaks on different cell cultures are not uniform and in part contradictory (Table 4).
The strong inhibition of break repair at higher concentrations provides no exact information in so far as Act. D, like bleomycin, induces breaks itself, which could mask the repair that have actually taken place. Only did Lee [44] observe on L1210 cells inhibi-

tion of single-strand rejoining at a very low concentration (0.028 μg/ml) which is approximately in the therapeutical dose range. The radiation intensifying effect of Act. D is interpreted by ELKIND such that the restitution of the DNA complex is prevented owing to the strong binding of Act. D with the DNA, because in his experiments on Chinese hamster cells radiation-induced DNA breaks were mended also in the presence of the substance.

Table 4. Influence of Actinomycin D on DNA Repair

Object	Concentration (μg/ml)	Inhibition of Repair	Type of Repair	Authors	
L5178Y cells	0.5	—	break rejoining (s)	SAWADA et al.	(1970)
mouse L cells	1.0	—	break rejoining (s)	TSUBOI et al.	(1970)
M. radiodurans	1.0	++	break rejoining (d)	KITAYAMA et al.	(1971)
L5178Y cells	0.1	—	break rejoining (s)	ORMEROD et al.	(1971)
Chin. hamster cells	6.3	—	break rejoining (s)	ELKIND et al.	(1972)
L1210 cells	0.7	++	break rejoining (s)	LEE et al.	(1972)
T cells	2.0	—	break rejoining (s)	KLEIJER et al.	(1973)
	20.0	++			
ascites hepatoma cells AM 66 F	5.0	+	break rejoining (bl)	MIYAKI et al.	(1973)
opossum lymphocytes		+	repair synthesis	MENEGHINI	(1974)
thymocytes of rat	1.0	+	break rejoining (s)	RYABCHENKO et al.	(1975)
mouse L5 cells	5.0	+	postreplication repair	FUJIWARA	(1975)

s single-strand breaks — no inhibition
d double-strand breaks + inhibition
bl bleomycin-induced breaks ++ complete inhibition

Caffeine

Caffeine (1,3,7-trimethylxanthine) as a purine derivative has been intensively studied for its mutagenic action and its influence on different intracellular recovery processes in various objects. The substance shows manifold effects on the genetic material both of normal and damaged bacterial and mammalian cell. Of special interest are studies on the influence of caffeine on lesions produced by UV-irradiation or alkylants, predominantly pyrimidine dimers [28, 58, 60, 74, 85, 93]. Since the capacity of radiationsensitive *E. coli* strains to effect pyrimidine dimer excision is limited, and caffeine shows here a much lower effect compared with the wild type, it has been inferred that caffeine exerts a direct inhibition on the excision process of dark repair [28, 60]. But since corresponding investigations on mammalian cells yielded conflicting results, the action mechanism of caffeine on repair events has yet to be elucidated. Thus, RAUTH [73] observed considerable effects of caffeine on the capacity of colony formation after UV-irradiation of L-cells of mouse. On the contrary, WILKINSON [106] using two different UV-sensitive HeLa cell lines and ARLETT [1] using Chinese hamster cells, were

unable to find a caffeine effect on the survival fraction of UV-irradiated mammalian cells, although here have been reported opposing results with regard to hamster cells [96, 97].
Proceeding from in vivo experiments on animal tumours in which the effect of radiation had been considerably increased by caffeine [22] and supposing that this effect was related to hindrance of repair processes, we studied in human tumour cells the influence of caffeine on the repair of DNA single-strand breaks following in vitro irradiation.
Figure 6 shows that caffeine (10^{-3} M) does not inhibit the repair of single-strand breaks in irradiated HeLa cells; corresponding results were obtained also in L5178Y-, T- and Chinese hamster cells [45, 41, 40].

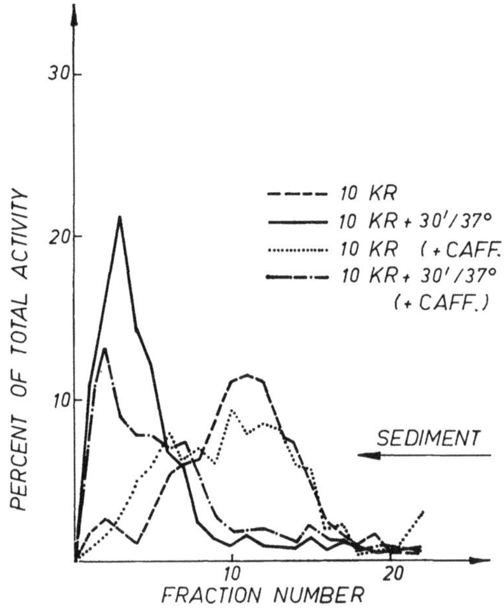

Fig. 6. DNA sedimentation profiles of irradiated and caffeine-treated HeLa cells (SCHRÖDER 1975).

Similarly, caffeine has no effects on the double-strand repair in HeLa- [102] and Chinese hamster cells and the nonsemiconservative DNA synthesis in the low doses range [8, 41]; in higher doses (100 krad) SEMENOVA et al. [87] found in HeLa cells suppression of the hydroxyurea-independent incorporation of ^{3}H TdR by caffeine. But there are numerous experimental results showing on various objects that caffeine specifically inhibits the postreplication repair [5, 10, 11, 18, 41, 46, 97], that is, it prevents in irradiated cells the low-molecular DNA synthesized shortly after irradiation from being transferred into a high-molecular form similar to the untreated controls.
The mechanism of caffeine sensibilization has been frequently discussed [5, 18, 45, 46, 82, 97] and is attributed basically to the addition of caffeine to the DNA or its influence on the enzymes involved in the DNA repair system.
A different possibility was proposed by LANG [42]. He assumes that caffeine causes reduction of the radiation-induced conformational change of DNA (C-form) into the

more stable B-form, as a result of which the structural changes of the DNA are no longer recognized by the enzymes involved in the repair process, and hence cannot be eliminated.

Hyperthermia

Especially prospective at the present time appears to be the combined tumour therapy including irradiation and simultaneous hyperthermia of the tumour area.
The revival of interest in hyperthermia in the last few years has prompted not only purely biological studies, but has exerted an influence on a number of molecularbiological topics. The few papers published so far on DNA repair processes under hyperthermic conditions justify the assumption that, up to ca. 42 °C, repair processes under oxic conditions are completely normal and are even partly intensified. Ben Hur [3] investigated the DNA repair of radiation-induced lesions under hyperthermic conditions on oxic Chinese hamster cells. He found out that after 6 krad the repair of DNA single-strand breaks up to 40 min post irradiation occurred faster at 42 °C than at 37 °C. After 10 krad the repair at 42 °C is no longer complete. Similarly, Ormerod et al. reported in 1971 [70] that the repair of DNA single-strand breaks is normal up to an incubation time of 40 min at elevated temperatures, after which the DNA is increasingly being degraded.
By contrast, the restitution of the DNA complex which is damaged already at low radiation doses but is required to keep the DNA functioning, is inhibited under hyperthermia [3].

Table 5. Temperature Optimum for the Repair of DNA Single-strand Breaks and the Unscheduled DNA Synthesis.

Cells	Radiation	Temperature Optimum (°C)		Authors
		SA	UDS	
lymphocytes	UV		42/44	Spiegler, Norman (1970)
lymphocytes	6 MeV electrons		40/42	Spiegler, Norman (1970)
lymphoma cells	ion. radiation	37 = 41/43		Ormerod, Stevens (1971)
Chin. hamster cells	ion. radiation	42		Ben Hur, Elkind (1974)
lymphoma cells	ion. radiation	42+		Schröder, Magdon (1977)
lymphocytes	ion. radiation		40/42	Schröder, Magdon (1977)

\+ = alkaline elution
SA = sedimentation analysis
UDS = unscheduled DNA synthesis

In experiments of our own we studied the temperature dependence of DNA repair in human normal lymphocytes and in lymphoma cells following irradiation with ^{60}Co in the temperature range from 37—44 °C. The results revealed an increase in thymidine incorporation up to 42° (Table 5). Further elevation of temperature causes a fall of unscheduled DNA synthesis below the normal value.

Similar results were obtained on lymphocytes by Spiegler and Norman [90] for the temperature optimum of unscheduled DNA synthesis induced by 6 MeV electrons.
The experiments with lymphoma cells were carried out by means of alkaline DNA elution [84]. The cell suspensions were irradiated respectively at 37 and 42° with 2 krad and immediately immersed in the ice-bath. Subsequent DNA elution showed that the eluation curves from samples irradiated at 42° were almost similar to those of the untreated control, i.e., the normalization processes occurring already during the irradiation must have occurred much faster at 42° than at 37°.
These studies have shown that raising the temperature up to 42° in cells well supplied with oxygen has no adverse effect on special repair mechanisms at the DNA, and may even reinforce them. It is likely that the hyperthermia-increased sensitiveness of some hypoxic tumour cells to irradiation is attributable to further inhibition of recovery processes which are already slowed under hypoxic conditions.
A critical review of the findings available at present shows that, although a broad variety of substances has been examined, the latter limit not only the DNA repair but also nucleic acid and protein synthesis almost. Therefore, future investigations should be aimed at finding substances with higher specificity of action and higher selectivity for tumour and normal cells.

References

[1] Arlett, C. F.: Int. J. Radiat. Biol. **13**, 369 (1967)
[2] Ben-Hur, E., Ben-Ishai, R.: Photochem.-biol. **13**, 337 (1971)
[3] Ben-Hur, E., Elkind, M. M.: Radiat. Res. **59**, 484 (1974)
[4] Bleehen, N. M., Gillies, N. E., Twentyman, P. R.: Brit. J. Radiol. **47**, 346 (1974)
[5] Buhl, St. N., Regan, J. D.: Biophys. J. **14**, 519 (1974)
[6] Byfield, J. E., Lee, Y. C., Tu, L., Kulhanian, F.: Cancer Res. **36**, 1138 (1976)
[7] Cabela, E., Klein, W.: Wien. Klin. W'schr. **88**, 299 (1976)
[8] Cleaver, J. E.: Radiat. Res. **37**, 334 (1969)
[9] Cleaver, J. E.: Radiat. Res. **37**, 428 (1969)
[10] Cleaver, J. E., Thomas, G. H.: Biochem. Biophys. Res. Commun. **36**, 203 (1969)
[11] Cleaver, J. E., Bootsma, D.: Ann. Rev. Genetics **9**, 19 (1975)
[12] Corry, P. M., Cole, A.: Radiat. Res. **36**, 528 (1968)
[13] Dalrymple, G. V., Sanders, J. L., Baker, M. L., Wilkinson, K. P.: Radiat. Res. **47**, 660 (1971)
[14] Dalrymple, G. V., Baker, M. L., Sanders, J. L., Moss, A. J., Nash, J. C., Wilkinson, K. P.: J. theoret. Biol. **28**, 121 (1971)
[15] Dean, C. J., Ormerod, M. G., Serianni, R. W., Alexander, P.: Nature **222**, 1042 (1969)
[16] Eberl, R., Tausch, G., Klein, W., Kocsis, F., Altmann, H.: Z. Rheumatol. **33**, 148 (1974)
[17] Elkind, M. M., Chang-Liu, C. M.: Int . J. Radiat. Biol. **22**, 313 (1972)
[18] Fujiwara, Y.: Biophys. J. **15**, 403 (1975)
[19] Fuks, Z., Smith, K. C.: Radiat. Res. **48**, 63 (1971)
[20] Ganesan, A. K., Smith, K. C.: J. Bacteriol. **111**, 575 (1972)
[21] Gaudin, D., Yielding, K. L.: Proc. Soc. Biol. Med. **131**, 1413 (1969)
[22] Gaudin, D., Yielding, K. L., Stabler, A., Brown, J.: Proc. Soc. Biol. Med. **137**, 202 (1971)
[23] Gaudin, D., Gregg, R. S., Yielding, K. L.: Proc. Soc. Biol. Med. **141**, 543 (1972)
[24] Gaudin, D., Gregg, R. S., Yielding, K. L.: Biochem. Biophys. Res. Commun. **45**, 630 (1971)
[25] Ginsberg, D. M., Webster, H. K.: Radiat. Res. **39**, 421 (1969)
[26] Grigg, G. W. J. Gen. Microbiol. **70**, 221 (1972)

[27] GRIGG, G. W., EDWARDS, M. J., BROWN, D. J.: J. Bacteriol. **107**, 599 (1971)
[28] HARM, W.: Mutation Res. **4**, 93 (1967)
[29] HARM, W.: Mutation Res. **10**, 319 (1970)
[30] HEMMEN, J. J. VAN, MEULING, W. J. A., JONG, J. DE, LUTHJENS, L. H.: Int. J. Radiat. Biol. **25**, 455 (1974)
[31] HORKAY, I., NAGY, E., TAMASI, P., SZABO, M., CSONGOR, J.: Studia biophys. **50**, 1 (1975)
[32] KAPP, D. S., SMITH, K. C.: Int. J. Radiat. Biol. **19**, 255 (1971)
[33] KITAYAMA, S., MATSUYAMA, A.: Agr. Biol. Chem. **35**, 644 (1971)
[34] KLEIN, G., WOTTAWA, A., ALTMANN, H., EBERL, R.: Arzneimittelforsch. **24**, 1975 (1974)
[35] KLEIN, G., WOTTAWA, A., ALTMANN, H.: Arzneimittelforsch. **25**, 288 (1975)
[36] KLEIN, G., WOTTAWA, A., ALTMANN, H., EBERL, R.: Wien. Klin. W'schr. **86**, 369 (1974)
[37] KLEIN, G., KOCSIS, F., EBERL, R., ALTMANN, H.: Z. Klin. Chem. Biochem., **12**, 75 (1974)
[38] KLEIN, G., ALTMANN, H., WOTTAWA, H., EBERL, R.: Arzneimittelforsch. **24**, 960 (1974)
[39] KLEIN, W., KOCSIS, F., EBERL, R., ALTMANN, H.: Studia biophys. **41**, 51 (1973)
[40] KLEIJER, K. J., HOEKSEMA, J. L., SLUYTER, M. L., BOOTSMA, D.: Mutation Res. **17**, 385 (1973)
[41] KÖRNER, I. J., MALZ, W., PITRA, CH.: Biol. Zbl. **95**, 561 (1976)
[42] LANG, H.: Studia biophys. **50**, 213 (1975)
[43] LANGENBACH, R., KUSZYNSKI, C. J.: J. Nat. Cancer Inst. **55**, 801 (1975)
[44] LEE, Y. CH., BENNETT, L. R., BYFIELD, J. E.: Biochem. biophys. Res. Commun. **49**, 758 (1972)
[45] LEHMANN, A. R.: Biophys. J. **12**, 1316 (1972)
[46] LEHMANN, A. R., KIRK-BELL, S., ARLETT, C. F., PATERSON, M. C., LOHMAN, P. H. M., WEERD-KASTELEIN, E. A. DE, BOOTSMA, D.: Proc. Nat. Acad. Sci. **72**, 219 (1975)
[47] LEWIS, N., KUMTA, U.: Radiat. Res. **62**, 159 (1975)
[48] LIEB, M.: Z. Vererbungslehre **92**, 416 (1961)
[49] LOHMAN, P. H. M., VOS, O., SLUIS, C. A. VAN, COHEN, J. A.: Biochim. Biophys. Acta **224**, 339 (1970)
[50] LOPEZ ZUMEL, M. C., ASTUDILLO, M. D., ALVAREZ, M. V.: Studia biophys. **50**, 107 (1975)
[51] MAGDON, E., SCHRÖDER, E., HIRSCH, G.: Strahlentherapie **127**, 282 (1965)
[52] MAGDON, E., SCHRÖDER, E.: Strahlentherapie **142**, 195 (1971)
[53] MAGDON, E., GUMMEL, H.: Dtsch. Gesundheitswes. **27**, 385 (1972)
[54] MAGDON, E.: Radioprotection and rejoining of DNA breaks, Vortrag, 10th Annual Meeting of the European Society for Radiation Biology, Madrid, 12.—13. 10. 1973
[55] MASKER, W. E.: Biochim. Biophys. Acta **442**, 162 (1976)
[56] MATSUDAIRA, H., FURUNO, I.: Biochim. Biophys. Acta **272**, 202 (1972)
[57] MAURICE, P. A., LEDERSEY, C.: Schweiz. med. W'schr. **104**, 149 (1974)
[58] MENDELSON, D.: Mutation Res. **22**, 145 (1974)
[59] MENEGHINI, R.: Chem. Biol. Interact. **8**, 113 (1974)
[60] METZGER, K.: Biochem. biophys. Res. Commun. **15**, 101 (1964)
[61] MICHAEL, R. O., WILLIAMS, G. M.: Mutation Res. **25**, 391 (1974)
[62] MIYAKI, M., MOROHASHI, S., ONO, T.: J. Antibiotics **26**, 369 (1973)
[63] MOSS, A. J., DALRYMPLE, G. V., SANDERS, J. L., WILKINSON, K. P., NASH, J. G.: Biophys. J. **11**, 158 (1971)
[64] MUKHERJEE, R., ALTMANN, H., IVANOVA, S.: Studia biophys. **50**, 117 (1975)
[65] MYERS, D. K.: Int. J. Radiat. Biol. **19**, 293 (1971)
[66] MYERS, D. K., CHETTY, K. G.: Radiat. Res. **53**, 307 (1973)
[67] NAIR, C. K. K., PRADHAN, D. S.: Int. J. Radiat. Biol. **29**, 235 (1976)
[68] NOGUTI, T., SADAIE, H., KADA, T.: Int. J. Radiat. Biol. **19**, 305 (1971)
[69] NOMURA, T.: Nature **260**, 547 (1976)
[70] ORMEROD, M. G., STEVENS, U.: Biochim. Biophys. Acta **232**, 72 (1971)

[71] PITRA, CH., HARTWIG, M., KÖRNER, I. J., MALZ, W.: Studia biophys. **62**, 31 (1977)
[72] RASMUSSEN, R. E.: Life Sciences **17**, 767 (1976)
[73] RAUTH, A. M.: Radiat. Res. **31**, 121 (1967)
[74] REGAN, J. D., TROSKO, J. E., CARRIER, W. L.: Biophys. J. **8**, 319 (1968)
[75] REVESZ, L., EDGREN, M., MODIG, H.: Studia biophys. **53**, 103 (1975)
[76] ROOTS, R., OKADA, S.: Int. J. Radiat. Biol. **21**, 329 (1972)
[77] RYABCHENKO, N. I., IVANNIK, B. P.: Studia biophys. **53**, 41 (1975)
[78] SASKA, J., NECASOVA, J.: Studia biophys. **36**, 259 (1973)
[79] SAWADA, S., OKADA, S.: Radiat. Res. **41**, 145 (1970)
[80] SAWADA, S., OKADA, S.: Radiat. Res. **44**, 116 (1970)
[81] SCHANS, G. P. VAN DER, BLOCK, J.: Int. J. Radiat. Biol. **17**, 25 (1970)
[82] SCHRÖDER, E., MAGDON, E.: Studia biophys. **51**, 209 (1975)
[83] SCHRÖDER, E., MAGDON, E.: Studia biophys. **61**, 151 (1977)
[84] SCHRÖDER, E., MAGDON, E.: Studia biophys. **64**, 193 (1977)
[85] SCHROY, C. B., TODD, P.: Mutation Res. **33**, 347 (1975)
[86] SCHUEREN, E. VAN DER, SMITH, K. C., KAPLAN, H. S.: Radiat. Res. **55**, 346 (1973)
[87] SEMENOVA, E. G., VOLKOVA, Z. M., ZHESTYANIKOV, V. D.: Zitologija **16**, 1010 (1974)
[88] SKARSGARD, L. D., PALCIC, B.: Int. J. Radiat. Biol. **21**, 535 (1972)
[89] SMITH, K. C.: Proc. XI. Int. Cancer Congr., Florence 1974, **5**, 105 (1975)
[90] SPIEGLER, P., NORMAN, A.: Radiat. Res. **43**, 187 (1970)
[91] STEHLIK, G., DELAC, M., KOHLWEIN, E.: Studia biophys. **50**, 151 (1975)
[92] SWEET, D. M., MOSELEY, B. E. B.: Mutation Res. **23**, 311 (1974)
[93] SWIETLIŃSKA, Z., ZUK, J.: Mutation Res. **26**, 89 (1974)
[94] TAUSCH, G., TUSCHL, P., DUNKY, A., EBERL, R.: Arzneimittelforsch. **25**, 291 (1975)
[95] TOWN, C. T., SMITH, K. C., KAPLAN, H. S.: In "Current Topics in Radiat. Res." **VIII**, 388 (1974)
[96] TROSKO, J. E., CHU, E. H. Y.: Mutation Res. **12**, 337 (1971)
[97] TROSKO, J. E., CHU, E. H. Y.: Chem.-Biol. Interactions **6**, 317 (1973)
[98] TROSKO, J. E., FRANK, P., CHU, E. H. Y.: Cancer Res. **33**, 2444 (1973)
[99] TSUBOI, A., TERASIMA, T.: Mol. Gen. Genet. **108**, 117 (1970)
[100] TUSCHL, P., KLEIN, W., KOCSIS, F., BERNAT, E., ALTMANN, H.: Environ. Physiol. Biochem. **5**, 84 (1975)
[101] TUSCHL, P., TAUSCH, G., EBERL, R.: Studia biophys. **50**, 172 (1975)
[102] VIKHANSKAIA, F. C., PINTO, R. I.: Dokl. Akad. Nauk SSSR **226**, 1436 (1976)
[103] VOICULETZ, N., SMITH, K. C., KAPLAN, H. S.: Cancer Res. **34**, 1038 (1974)
[104] VOICULETZ, N., SBENGHE, M., SANDULESCU, T.: Studia biophys. **50**, 97 (1975)
[105] WALDSTEIN, E. A., SHARON, R., BEN-ISHAI, R.: Proc. Nat. Acad. Sci. **71**, 2651 (1974)
[106] WILKINSON, R., KIEFER, J., NIAS, H. A. W.: Mutation Res. **10**, 67 (1970)
[107] YIELDING, L. W., RILEY, T. L., YIELDING, K. L.: Biochem. biophys. Res. Commun. **68**, 1356 (1976)

Photodynamically Induced DNA Damage, their Repair and the Influence of Different Chemicals on the Repair Process

H.-E. Jacob

Akademie der Wissenschaften der DDR
Zentralinstitut für Mikrobiologie und experimentelle Therapie
Abteilung Biophysikochemie, 69 Jena, Beuthenbergstraße 11

The components of photodynamic action are light (in the range from 400 to 700 nm), a sensitizer (in general substances absorbing in the range of visible light = dyes), oxygen, and the object which should be changed. The photodynamic action is the result of a sensitized photochemical oxydation, and in general the objects are molecules (i.e. aminoacids (Jori et al. 1969), proteins (Spikes and Livingston 1969), RNA and DNA) or living cells (i.e. bacteria, algae (Raab 1900)). Using living cells the photodynamic

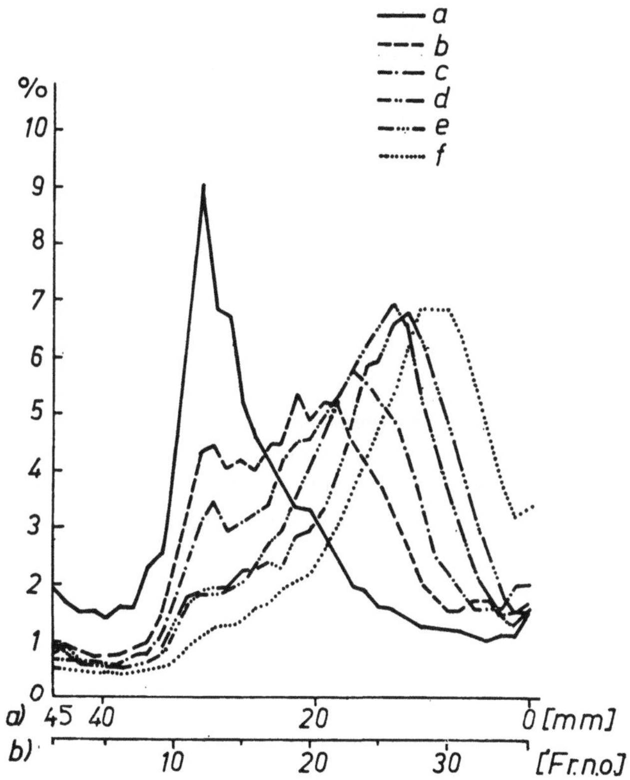

Fig. 1. Changes in the sedimentation pattern of single-strandes DNA from *P. mirabilis* VI PG 273 treated photodynamically (visible light, methylene blue, air).

a non-illuminated
b 5 s illuminated
c 15 s illuminated
d 30 s illuminated
e 60 s illuminated
f 180 s illuminated

action results in a killing, this means a decrease of survivors. The degree of killing depends on the dye used and their concentration, on the illumination time with visible light and the output of the lamp.
The action of the photodynamic effect on several biomolecules i.e. proteins and nucleic acids has been studied in the last 15 years. In nucleic acids the photodynamic action destroys guanine (Simon and van Vunakis 1962, Wacker et al. 1963). The investigations of Sastry and Gordon (1966) showed that photodynamic treatment of guanosine, besides producing alterations in the guanine part, may also result in the breakage of the N-glycosidic bond between guanine and deoxyribose. In DNA the apurinic sites resulting from this are unstable in the presence of alkali (Tamm et al. 1953) and give rise to single-strand breaks. Further evidence that one target of the photodynamic action is the DNA results from investigations with mutants of bacterial strains. As Böhme (1968), Böhme and Geissler (1968), and Harm (1968) have shown, there are differences in the survival of *Proteus mirabilis* and *Escherichia coli* between "wild-type" and *hcr rec* mutant strains after photodynamic action. — If there are changes in the DNA resulting in apurinic sites it should be possible to detect this by centrifugation, because such apurinic sites give rise to single-strand breaks under alkaline conditions.
Some results of investigations by means of alkaline sucrose gradients using ^3H labelled DNA (Jacob 1971) are shown in Fig. 1. We measure single-strand breaks, but these measurements do not allow one to decide whether the DNA single-strand breaks are caused directly by the photodynamic action, or secondarily by the alkaline treatment, or both.
Independently from this, the method is useful in studying repair processes after photodynamic inactivation of cells. If during repair time a decrease in the number of single-strand breaks is measurable, then repair on the DNA has taken place.

Methods

The methods used in general are not given here. They are published elsewhere (Jacob 1971, 1975). It must be mentioned here that the representation of the results of the experiments is given by the position of the center of gravity. This value is computed from the measurements in the liquid scintillation counter by means of a special programme.

Result and discussion

At first some remarks on the kinetics of the sedimentation behavior of DNA during photodynamic treatment. The results obtained with two strains of *P. mirabilis* VI PG 273 (wild-type) and PG 672 (*rec*$^-$) are shown in Fig. 2. It can be seen from this convenient index of sedimentation behavior that in both PG 273 and PG 672 the changes in sedimentation of DNA are nearly the same. In both strains the sedimentation velocity decreases most rapidly immediately after start of illumination. However, the number of survivors in the two strains is different with the surviving fraction being distinctly lower in strain PG 672 at a given dose.

An important observation was that photodynamic treatment of bacteria resulted in a decrease of the amount of "sediment" collected from the bottom of the tubes. In the non-treated control (100% survival) 14% of the radioactivity is sedimented. At a survival rate of 25% the "sediment" however contains only 4% of the total counts. It

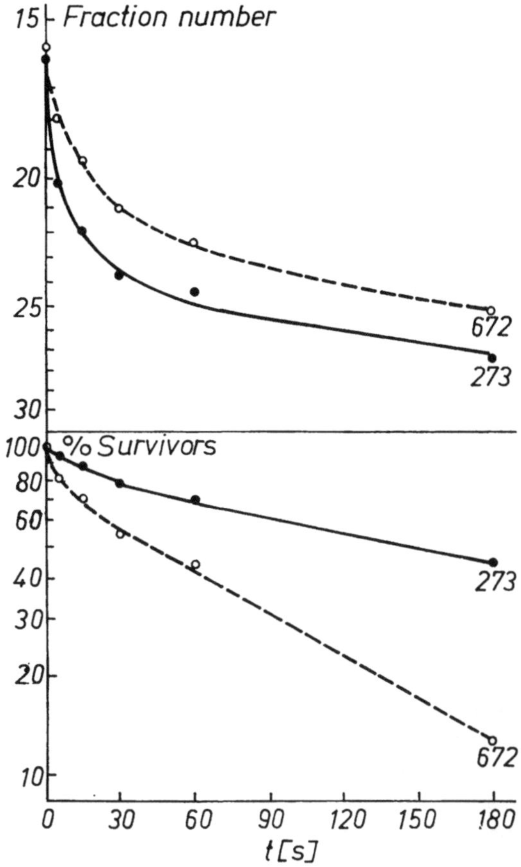

Fig. 2. Photodynamic action on the two strains PG 273 and PG 672.
a) Changes in the sedimentation behavior of single-stranded DNA (position of the center of gravity)
b) survival

should be mentioned here that photodynamic treatment changes the cell envelope and these changes are reparable, too (Jacob and Hamann 1975).
The results of typical experiments about repair of DNA damage with strain PG 273 are presented in Fig. 3: As shown before, photodynamic treatment reduced the sedimentation velocity of DNA. After illumination the sedimentation rate of DNA increases. In the case of low killing (Fig. 3a) a sedimentation profile similar to that of the reference sample is obtained after 20 min of incubation. In the case of strong killing the amount of damaged DNA is high and the recognition of repair processes is difficult be-

cause the repaired fraction is below the level of detection. Curves b and c of Fig. 3 show experimental results carried out at intermediate levels of inactivation.
After photodynamic inactivation, the repair processes of strain PG 273 are finished in about 20 min. Prolonged time in nutrient medium does not lead to further repair, but the radioactivity of the layered lysate decreases, lysis of the cells is more difficult, and the amount of "sediment" increases. Finally, after about 40 min an increase in the number of cells, resulting from normal cell division, could be detected.

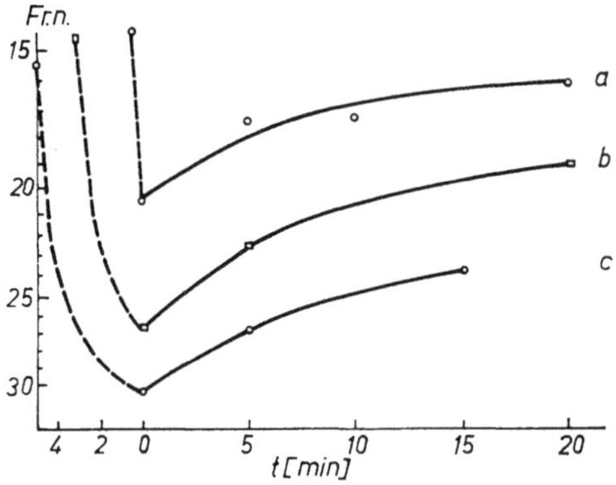

Fig. 3. In viro repair of photodynamically damaged DNA as a function of inactivation (*P. mirabilis* VI PG 273).

Repair experiments carried out at 37° and at 0 °C clearly demonstrate the temperature dependence of the repair process since no repair was observed during incubation at 0 °C for 20 min. — When the cells were incubated in the borate buffer for 20 min at 37 °C no repair of photodynamic damage in DNA took place.
Experiments with strain PG 672 show a very small repair only at a low inactivation. At a higher inactivation no repair occurs (see Fig. 4). The necessity of 10 min incubation time between drawing the sample and pipetting it on the gradient (time of lysis) should not influence the sedimentation profile (see results with strain PG 273).

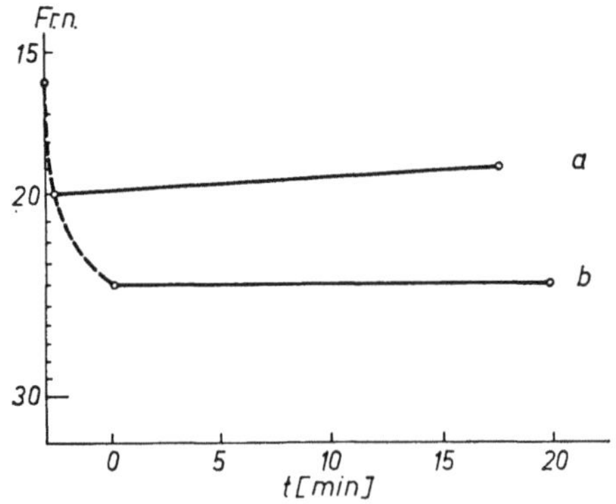

Fig. 4. In viro repair of photodynamically damaged DNA as a function of inactivation (*P. mirabilis* VI PG 672).

As a substance inhibiting the repair after UV inactivation caffeine is well known. With *P. mirabilis* VI PG 273 the action of caffeine was studied by K. STÖRL and the presence of this chemical compound in the repair medium did virtually not result in any repair of UV produced DNA damage. On the contrary after photodynamic treatment no differences arise between the samples with or without caffeine.
Another repair inhibitor is quinacrine (QA). FUKS and SMITH (1971) studied the repair inhibition after X-ray inactivation of bacteria. In *rec*$^+$ strains of *E. coli* 1.5×10^{-4} M/l QA resulted in a strong inhibition of repair, measured by means of the sucrose gradient technique. But QA has a considerable dark effect and resulting from this the surviving fraction shows a decrease. *Rec* 13 mutants do not exhibit any effect of QA; these mutants lack a repair system for X-irradiation and they are much more sensitive to X-ray than the wild-type bacteria. The same inhibiting effect was observed in eucaryotic cells (VOICULETZ et al. 1974). Because the repair of photodynamic damage produced with acridine-orange depends on the *rec* and *hcr* systems (HARM 1968), this substance should act as an inhibitor. And in our experiments QA addition to the repair medium results in the expected manner: QA acts as an inhibitor of DNA repair after photodynamic treatment.
From the results obtained with these repair inhibitors we get further information that there is a difference between the repair of DNA lesions produced by UV-irradiation on the one hand and by X-ray and by photodynamic treatment on the other, and that two different systems must work for the repair of these damages. The results reported here are in good agreement with the phenotypic characteritation of the *P. mirabilis* strains examined, too.
If acriflavine (AF) is used as substance an inhibition of the repair of photodynamic DNA damage takes place. As well as with QA there is a considerable decrease in the number of survivors. From *E. coli* HARM (1973) reported that AF in concentrations $> 1.2 \times 10^{-5}$ M/l in the repair medium inhibited the *hcr* system completely. That AF inhibits the repair of DNA damage in Xeroderma pigmentosum cells brought about by X-ray was published by KLEIJER et al. (1973). These results show in respect of the repair inhibition the same tendency as caffeine and QA. But some more experimental data must be available, especially in the field of UV inactivation.
The investigations with compounds, used by several authors for inhibition of repair, served in our experiments as a tool for distinguishing the different repair systems in bacteria.

Summary

These investigations are examining DNA repair of strains of *P. mirabilis* VI after photodynamic inactivation. Sedimentations experiments with alkaline sucrose gradient technique allow the following conclusions:

1) A given dose of illumination induces approximately the same amount of initial damages in the DNA of the repair-proficient strain PG 273 and of the sensitive mutant PG 672.
2) Repair of photodynamic damage of DNA can be demonstrated with strain PG 273 in growth medium at 37 °C. The repair depends on temperature; complete inhibition takes place at 0 °C. — In strain PG 672 only a slight repair was seen.

3) The time necessary for repair is about 20 min.
4) With the repair inhibitors caffeine (C), quinacrine (QA), and acriflavine (AF) after photodynamic DNA damage we observed:
   a) C does not inhibit the repair. C acts only on UV produced damage
   b) QA has the same inhibitora effect as described for repair of DNA after X-ray treatment
   c) AF inhibits the repair. AF is also an inhibitor of repair after X-ray. Further investigations using AF must be done, especially in the field of UV-inactivation.

References

BÖHME, H.: Mutation Res. **6**, 166—168 (1968)

BÖHME, H., GEISSLER, E.: Mol. Genetics **103**, 228—232 (1968)

FUKS, Z., SMITH. K. C.: Radiation Res. **48**, 63—73 (1971)

HARM, W.: Biochem. Biophys. Res. Commun. **32**, 350—358 (1968)

HARM, W.: Mutation Res. **17**, 163—176 (1973)

JACOB, H.-E.: Photochem. Photobiol. **14**, 743—745 (1971)

JACOB, H.-E.: Photochem. Photobiol. **21**, 445—447 (1975)

JACOB, H.-E., HAMANN, M. (1975): Photochem. Photobiol. (in press)

JORI, G., GALIAZZO, G., SCOFFONE, E.: Biochemistry 8, 2868—2875 (1969)

KLEIJER, W. J., HOEKSEMA, J. L., SLUYTER, M. L., BOOTSMA, D.: Mutation Res. **17**, 385—394 (1963)

RAAB, O.: Z. Biol. **39**, 524—531 (1900)

SASTRY, K. S., GORDON, M. P.: Biochim. Biophys. Acta **129**, 42—48 (1966)

SIMON, M. I., VAN VUNAKIS, H.: J. Mol. Biol. **4**, 488—499 (1962)

SPIKES, J. D., LIVINGSTON, R.: Adv. Radiat. Biol. **3**, 29—121 (1969)

STÖRL, K. personal communication

TAMM, C. H., SHAPPIRO, H. S., LIPSCHITZ, R., CHARGAFF, E.: J. Biol. Chem. **203**, 673—688 (1953)

VOICULETZ, N., SMITH, K. C., KAPLAN, H. S.: Cancer Res. **34**, 1038—1044 (1974)

WACKER, A., TÜRK, G., GERSTENBERGER, A.: Naturwissenschaften **50**, 377 (1963)

An Influence of Freezing the Cells on the Formation of Single-Strand Breaks in DNA after Irradiation

Jurášková V., Drášil V.

Institute of Biophysics, Czechoslovak Academy of Sciences, Brno

Radiosensitivity of mammalian cells varies over a wide range in dependence on the conditions of irradiation. Our previous experiments have shown that a significant increase in the D_0 dose occurs if cells are irradiated in frozen state. The D_0 value was raised up to 600—800 rads if cells were irradiated at temperatures of -74 °C and -196 °C (Drášil and Jurášková 1964).
In the present study damage and repair processes in the DNA at these conditions were followed using velocity sedimentation in alkaline sucrose gradients.

Material and methods

In our experiments Ehrlich ascites tumour cells labeled overnight with tritiated thymidine were used. The freezing of cells was carried out in the presence of glycerol (15%) or dimethylsulphoxide (7%). The rate of cooling was about 1°C per min to -20 °C and then the cells were transferred into Dry Ice or liquid nitrogen. Cells were irradiated while suspended by γ-rays of ^{60}Co at an exposure rate of 1.500 rads per min. The survival curves were obtained by counting the cells in the peritoneal cavity of mice on the fourth day after the injection of a constant size inoculum.

Results

In Table 1 values of D_0 and extrapolation numbers for EAT cells irradiated under different conditions can be seen. The D_0 value is raised from 118 rads under irradiation at room temperature up to about 700 rads under irradiation at frozen state.

Table 1. EAT Cells Irradiated at Different Conditions.

Temperature during Irradiation	Irradiated in Presence of	Do rad	n
+20 °C	O_2	118	2.9
	N_2	345	6.3
−74	O_2	325	2.9
	N_2	790	3.0
−196	O_2	692	3.8
	N_2	780	3.4

Figure 1 shows the relationship between DNA injury and the concentration of glycerol at two temperatures: 0 °C and -196 °C. Ionizing radiation produced one single-strand break in the DNA of mammalian cells per energy absorption of 40—70 eV. This value is raised to less than 130 eV at the temperature of —196 °C, the concentration of glycerol in the medium being 15%.

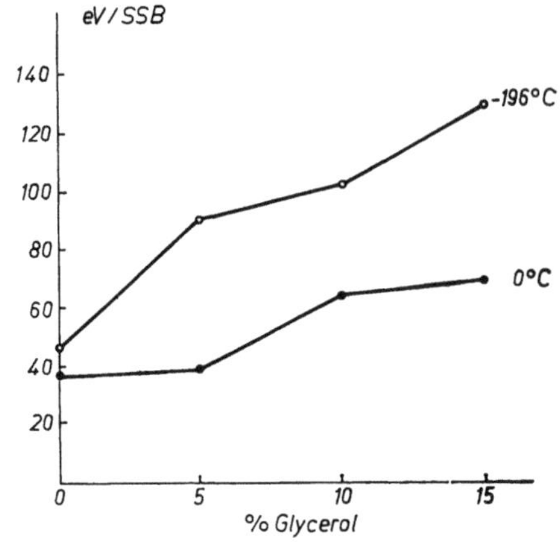

Fig. 1. The dependence of energy required for induction of ssb on the concentration of glycerol.
○—○—: irradiated at 0 °C; ●—●—: irradiated at —196 °C.

The sedimentation profile of the DNA from EAT cells irradiated with a dose of 10.000 rads is shown in Fig. 2. Curve No. 1 (open circles) in this figure was obtained by centrifugation of a control suspension of cells, i.e., cells which were irradiated at —196 °C and

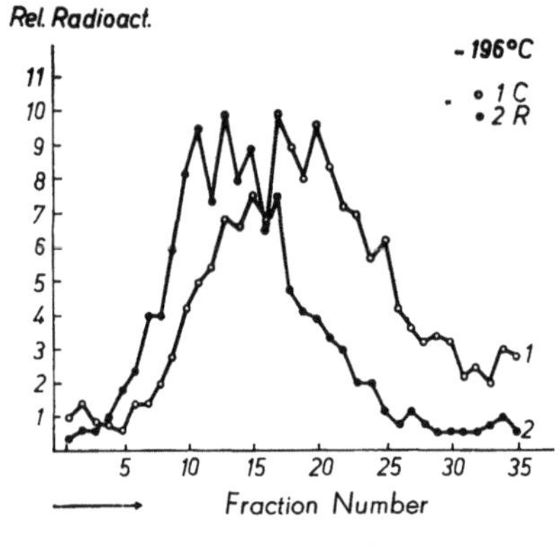

Fig. 2. Distribution of molecular weight of DNA of EAT cells irradiated at —196 °C.
○—○—○: no incubation after irradiation
●—●—●: 60 min incubation after irradiation

transferred on top of sucrose gradient immediately after thawing. Curve No. 2 (closed circles) shows the distribution of molecular weights of the DNA from cells irradiated at —196 °C and incubated in the nutrient medium after thawing for a period of 60 min. A shift to lower molecular weight values is obvious from the figure. Thus no ssb repair and increase in molecular weight were observed during incubation. Analogous results were obtained also when cells were cooled to a temperature of —74 °C.

Figure 3 illustrates the results of experiments in which the ability to synthesize the DNA in EAT (by means of ^{3}H-thymidine incorporation) was followed in the cells after freezing and thawing. It is apparent that this ability remains practically uninfluenced by freezing to temperatures of up to −74 °C. Upon a decrease in temperature to −196 °C, cells do not incorporate ^{3}H-thymidine into the DNA measurable quantities after thawing.

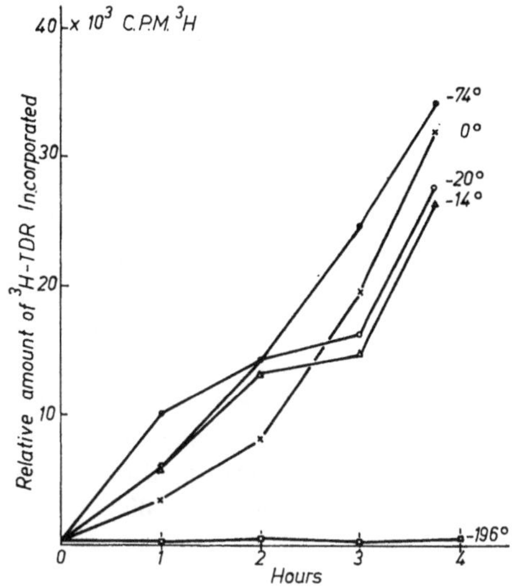

Fig. 3. The DNA synthesis in EAT cells after freezing and thawing at various temperatures.

Cells were frozen to: x—x—: 0 °C; △—△—: −14 °C; ○—○—: −20 °C; ●—●—: −74 °C; □—□—: −196 °C

Discussion

Exposure to low temperatures damages cells and alters their biological function. Having centered our attention on the induction and rejoining of single-strand DNA breaks after irradiation of cells at frozen state, we have found that the ability of repair single-strand breaks is influenced considerably more by freezing than the ability to synthesize DNA. When cooling EAT cells to −196 °C we have not observed any further synthesis of DNA in the first hours after thawing. On the other hand, the survival rate of frozen — thawed cells in the presence of additives like glycerol or dimethylsulphoxide was about 20—35%. On the basis of our results we cannot yet conclude whether DNA synthesis would be subsequently restored in cells surviving freezing to −196 °C, or whether the freezing would be survived by cells which are in the presynthetic phase.

In view of the above mentioned results it could follow that single-strand breaks are not closely related to cell killing by radiation. It is well documented by a six-fold rise of D_0 values after irradiation at −196 °C on the one hand, and by only a three-fold decrease in the amount of single-strand breaks in DNA under same conditions of irradiation on the other hand. According to our results, the repair of single-strand breaks in the DNA after irradiation of cells at frozen state does not correlate with changes in radiosensitivity of cells, for the repair mechanism does not work in the first hours after thawing. When summarizing our results we can assume that there is probably no direct relationship between the formation of breaks in the DNA and their postirradiation repair and the cell recovery. Cleaver and his coworkers (Cleaver et al. 1972) observed in frozen Chinese hamster cells no alterations in repair of ssb after thawing. The difference between these and our results just described could be explained either by the rate of temperature decrease or by the different kind of cells.

Summary

Ehrlich ascites tumour cells were irradiated with gamma radiation (7500—22500 rad) at very low temperatures (—196 °C). Centrifugation in alkaline sucrose gradient was used for following the amount of single-strand breaks in DNA of the irradiated cells.
The results of the experiments showed that the amount of energy needed for one ssb on irradiating the frozen cells was approximately 46 eV, and was only by 30% higher than that found on irradiating the cells at 0 °C. Addition of glycerol (15% v.v.) to the suspension leads to an increase of the value given above to 130 eV. For the non-frozen cells the increase in the presence of glycerol is relatively lower, from 36 to 69 eV. If the irradiated cells are incubated in a nutrition medium after thawing, no repair of the single-strand breaks induced in the DNA by radiation can be observed. Also DNA synthesis is interrupted in spite of the fact that the suspension contains 20—35% of cells capable of multiplication.

Zusammenfassung

Die Ehrlich-Ascites-Tumorzellen wurden bei sehr niedrigen Temperaturen (—196 °C) gammabestrahlt (7500 bis 22500 R). Zur Verfolgung der Anzahl einsträngiger DNA-Brüche der bestrahlten Zellen wurde die Zentrifugierung im alkalischen Saccharosengradient angewandt.
Die Versuchsergebnisse ergaben daß die für einen einsträngigen Bruch bei Bestrahlung tiefgekühlter Zellen benötigte Energiemenge annähernd gleich 46 eV war, und somit bloß um 30% höher als dieselbe bei Bestrahlung von Zellen bei 0 °C ermittelte Menge war. Die Zugabe von Glyzerin (15%) in die Suspension führt zu einer Erhöhung des oben angegebenen Wertes auf 130 eV. Die Erhöhung bei nichttiefgekühlten Zellen in Anwesenheit von Glyzerin ist verhältnismäßig geringer, von 36 bis zu 69 eV. Sind die bestrahlten Zellen nach Auftauen in einem Nährmedium inkubiert, so kann keine Reparation der durch Bestrahlung in der DNA induzierten einsträngigen Brüche beobachtet werden. Gleichfalls die DNA-Synthese wird unterbrochen trotzdem, daß in der Suspension 20 bis 35% multiplikationsfähige Zellen enthalten sind.

Влияние замораживания на возникновение одиночных разрывов в ДНК после облучения

В работе были исследованы клетки асцитной опухоли Эрлиха при гамма облучении при низких температурах (—196 °C). Методом скоростной седиментации в алкалическом градиенте сахарозы устанавливалось количество одиночных разрывов в ДНК облученых клеток.

Результаты опытов показали, что количество энергии нужной для возникновения одного разрыва в облученой и замораживанной клетке приблизительно 46 eV. Если в среде находится глицерол повышается эта данная на 130 eV.
Установлено также что инкубация при 37 °C в течении 60 минут после облучения (замораживанных и оттаиванных клеток) не приводила восстановление разрывов в ДНК.

References

[1] Drášil, V., Jurášková, V.: Folia Biol., **10**, 366 (1964)
[2] Cleaver, J. E., Thomas, G. H., Burki, H. J.: Science, **177**, 996 (1972)

DISEASES ASSOCIATED WITH DEFECTIVE DNA REPAIR

Xeroderma Pigmentosum — Report of Three Cases and Ultrastructural Investigation of Sun-unexposed Tumour-free Skin

U.-F. HAUSTEIN, K. KLUGE and H. MEFFERT

Dept. Dermatology (Head: Prof. Dr. U.-F. HAUSTEIN) of the Karl-Marx-University of Leipzig, GDR

Dept. Dermatology (Head: Prof. Dr. E. GÜNTHER) of the Friedrich-Schiller-University of Jena, GDR

Dept. Dermatology (Head: Prof. Dr. N. SÖNNICHSEN) of the Humboldt-University of Berlin, GDR

Since KAPOSI first described Xeroderma pigmentosum (X.p.) in 1870, numerous synonyms have been used, e. g. senilitas cutis praecox, light shrinked skin ("Lichtschrumpfhaut"), epithéliomatose pigmentaire, carcinomatosis multiplex hereditaria [19]. The disorder is of an autosomal-recessive, rarely of autosomal-dominant heredity [12, 19, 34]. It is characterized by a typical light-sensitivity which leads to alterations at first of the light-exposed and later also of the unexposed parts of the skin. Generally the disease begins in an acute way in the first weeks or months of life, but it may also begin gradually during the first years and is followed by a relatively slow progression [31]. The tardaform which begins in adolescence is a rare one. Concerning the clinical course four stages of cutaneous changes can be differentiated [12, 19].

1. A preleminary stage of erythema formation which occurs recurrently as light induced inflammation and results in diffuse pigmentation. This stage may be omitted.
2. The stage of poikiloderma with vesicle formation, occurence of freckle-like spots, atrophies, teleangiectasias, angiomas, ectropium and conjunctivitis.
3. Precancerous stage with tense atrophy, actinic keratoses and superficial ulcerations.
4. The stage of tumour formation with basal cell epitheliomas, squamous cell carcinomas, malignant melanomas, sarcomas, including metastases [18].

A distinct condition is represented by the de Sanctis Cacchione Syndrome, the combination of the above mentioned skin alterations with proportionate dwarfism, oligophrenia, speech disorder, disturbance of coordination and neurologic reflexes, genital hypoplasia and occasionally abnormalities in porphyric metabolism.

Many of these patients die by tumour metastases, cachexia, and other secondary afflictions before the age of 20. Throughout their life they are isolated and psychically stressed. The therapy consists of protection from sunlight and continious medical observation in view to early diagnosis and treatment of the developing malignancies.

In this paper case reports are given of 3 patients with X.p. Further it is reported about the ultrastructural changes in four different areas of sun-unexposed tumour-free skin from one of the patients. The degree of the developement of the compulsory precancerous dermatosis is outlined, which in the sun-unexposed areas covered by clothes only seldom leads to the formation of the malignancies, but gives the possibility of histopathogenetic conclusions and comparisons with the light exposed skin.

Report of Cases:

The *first patient* (Berlin) was a girl who died at the age of 12 [see also ref. No. 23]. The parents were kin. At the age of 9 months after UV-irradiation an erythema of the face developed which persisted for some days and shaded into brownish freckles. During the summer months of the following years macular erythema and yellowish to darkbrown dense freckle-like pigmentations developed on the uncovered skin of face, neck, and back of the hands. Besides circumscribed whitish atrophies, numerous teleangiectasias, and some warty hyperkeratoses occurred. At the age of 3 1/2 a tumour developed in the right inner eye angle. Histological examination revealed an anaplastic squamous cell carcinoma, but in some areas structures resembling to a malignant melanoma were visible. This tumour and further developing malignancies were treated with Choul x-ray irradiation and Radium-application. At the age of 5 1/2 an ulcerated tumour had formed which extended from the right inner lid angle to the nares (Fig. 1a) and proved to be a squamous cell carcinoma. The skin of the face was covered with brown and black spots, small scars, and numerous verrucous hyperkeratoses. Nape and the backs of the hands were less intensively involved. The regions normally covered by clothes were without pathological changes except some dark pigmented naevi.
Laboratory Findings: The blood sedimentation rate was always moderately increased. The sensitivity to UV-radiation was considerably increased by both mercury radiation and xenon radiation source. In these investigations could be noted that the erythemas in the testing areas were fully developed only after 48 hours, they persisted up to one week, and the resulting hyperpigmentation was still visible after some months. The other laboratory studies showed no abnormality, there was no sign of liver damage or disturbed porphyric metabolism.

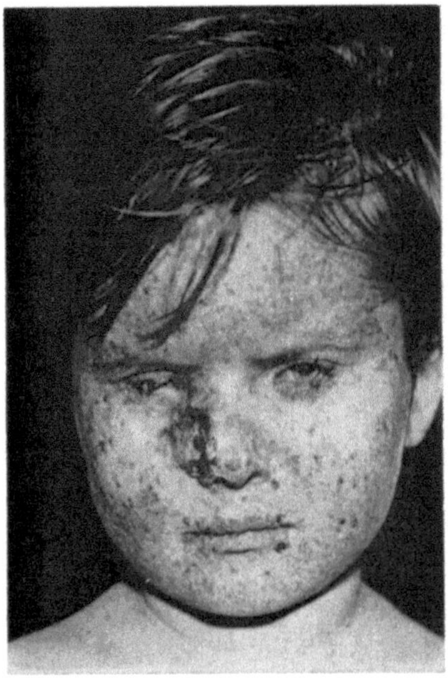

Fig. 1a

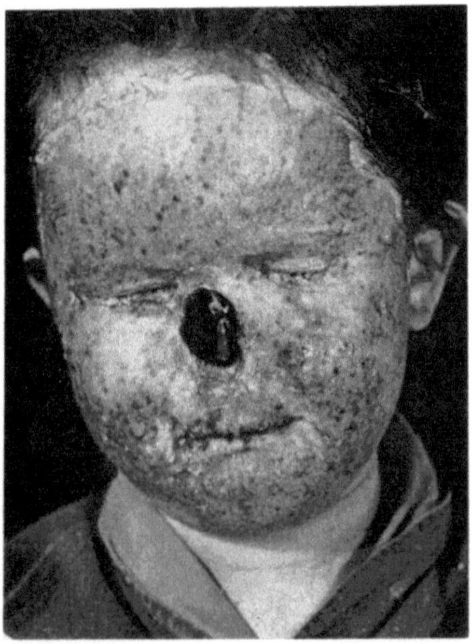

Fig. 1b

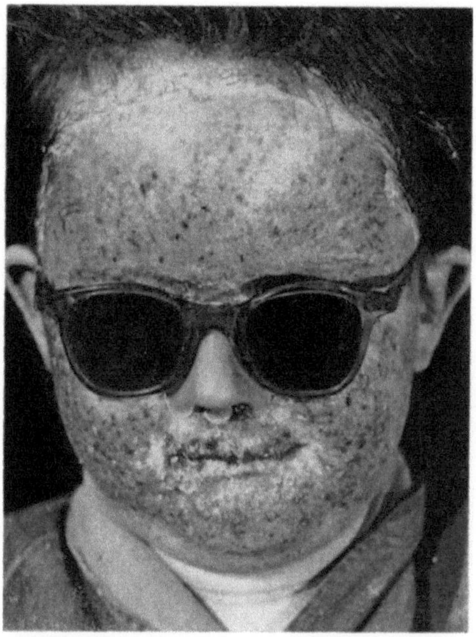

Fig. 1c

Fig. 1. a) 5-year-old girl (1rst patient) with squamous cell carcinoma of the nose. b) and and c) The same girl after amputation of the nose (b) and with epithetic repair (c). Note the scarred poikilodermatic skin.

The *therapy* consisted of surgical removal and x-ray irradiation of the malignant tumours which occured in steadily shortened intervals during the course of disease. Thus the excision of a necrotizing squamous cell carcinoma required the ablatio nasi (Fig. 1b). An epithesis brought about a good cosmetic result (Fig. 1c). The smaller tumours were removed by electrosurgery. The light-exposed skin was covered with paste, the child had to stay inside the house all day. The neoplasias were only located on face, neck and hands even during the latest months of her life. Despite the permanent supervision removal of the basal epitheliomas and squamous cell carcinomas, the general status deteriorated continously in her 11th year of life; she died at the age of 12.

The *2nd patient* (Jena) is a 22-year-old female (clerk), whose parents are not kin to each other. Increasing obesity, hypertension, chronic recurrent pyelonephritis, liability to infections of the upper respiratory tract have existed since 1967, additionally diabetes mellitus since 1970.

Already in her first year of life impressive large and dark freckles appeared on the light exposed areas of the integument besides photophobia. At the age of 3 first teleangiectasias, at age 4 the first wart-like skin alterations with haemorrhagic crusts occured on the face. During the next years the skin became more reddened and swollen with formation of pityriasiform scales, warty hyperkeratoses, mottled hyperpigmentations, and teleangiectasias (Fig. 2a).

The *treatment* was carried out with Chloroquine, later with vitamin A and E and Reducdyn(R). Locally Sulfathiazol PÄO I(R) and Contralum(R) were applied as sun screen. The hyperkeratoses were treated with Colchicin application and especially on the limbs they were removed mechanically. Since 1969 2,5% 5-Fluoro-uracil-preparations have been applied twice a year, since 1976 an attempt of β-Carotene medication by intake of carrot juice has been made. Numerous larger tumours were excised surgically and proved to be epidermal, mesenchymal, and pigmentforming neoplasias (Tab. 1). They were mainly located in the face, nape, lateral neck, upper side of the forearms, back of the hands and lower legs.

Table 1. Synopsis of the tumours of the second and the third patient (see fig. 4 to 11)

diagnosis	number of tumours	
	2nd patient	3rd patient
basal cell epithelioma	14	35
mixed carcinoma	6	3
squamous cell carcinoma	17	7
actinic keratosis	40	18
keratoakanthoma	2	4
haemangioma	9	17
granuloma pyogenicum	—	5
angiokeratoma	—	1
(angio) fibroma	—	4
histiocytoma	3	1
naevus-cell-naevus	3	1
lentigo benigna	1	—
melanosis praeblastomatosa Dubreuilh	6	4

Since 1972 the frequency of tumour formation has decreased (mean of 4 excisions per year compared with a mean of 10 excisions in the years before). In addition, the scaling and formation of warty hyperkeratoses are less pronounced, the integument is of an atrophic appearance; vascularization and mottled hyperpigmentation predominate (Fig. 2b, c). 50% of the neoplasias were haemangiomas and melanosis praeblastomatosa whereas before 1972 about 90% of all excised tumours were of epidermal origin. The very conscientious patient consequently avoids sun light and wears sun glasses.

Dermatological findings at present: The skin of the whole face looks very thin and tense so that many teleangiectasias are visible which partly form lentil-shaped tumours (Fig. 2d). On the neck, arms, back of the hands and lower legs the atrophy is less pronounced than in the face and decreases towards the trunk. On the trunk and the almost non-exposed thighs freckle-like hyperpigmentations of various intensities on otherwise unaltered integument are visible, decreasing in number and pigmentation from cranially to caudally on the trunk, upward on the thighs. Only on the buttocks and the abdomen from the girdle to the inguinal region ("site of the bathing shorts"), the skin is without pathological changes. The lanugo hair of the face has vanished, only in the less altered regions it is normal.

Ophthalmological finding: Madarosis of the upper lids, scarred ectropium formation of the lower lids with loss of the cilia; conjunctival reddening.

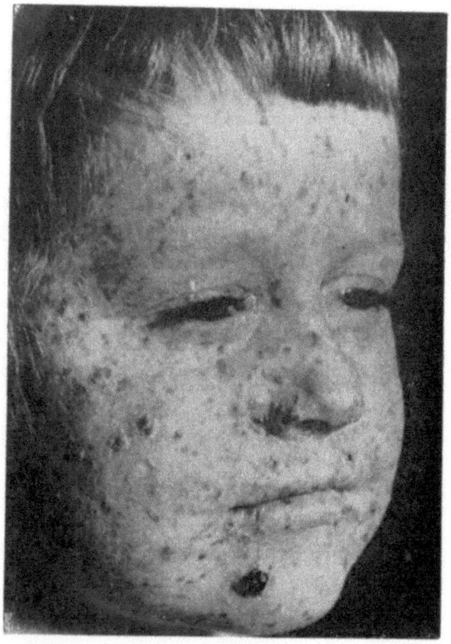

Fig. 2a

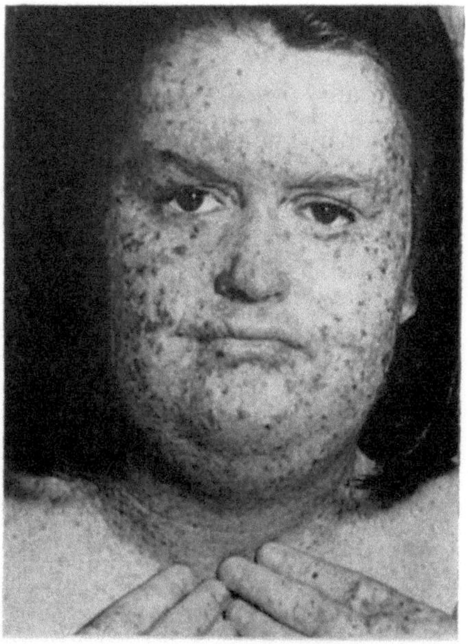

Fig. 2b

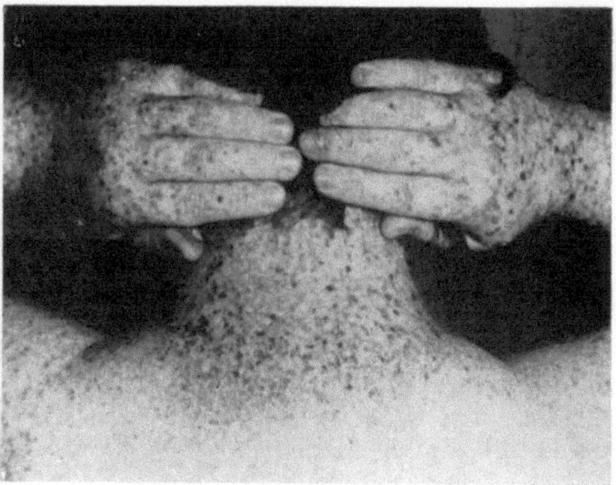

Fig. 2c

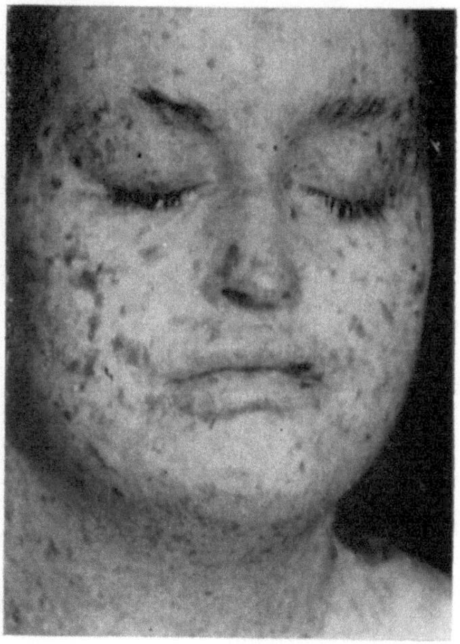

Fig. 2d

Fig. 2. a) 6-year-old girl (2nd patient) with several precancerous actinic keratoses, basaliomas and one haemangioma on the chin. b) The same girl at the age of 12. Note the impairment of the skin with several tumours and teleangiectasias. c) The same situation on the neck and back sides of the hands and fingers. d) 22 years old. The skin is predominantly scarred and atrophic. Numerous teleangiectasias and haemangiomas are evident.

Laboratory findings: β-Carotene level i.s. 75 γ/100 ml before initiation of Carrot-juice-therapy (normal); examination for DNA-antibodies, spontaneous UV-fluorescence of erythrocytes and skin specimens, abnormal secretion of porphyrines: negative.
UV-irradiations of the light-unexposed skin (Department of Dermatology, University of Greifswald): They were performed in the wave lengths between 260 nm and 500 nm (10 nm steps distances, in each series uniform radiation time for all wave lengths). The differences in the reactions elicited under identical conditions between the patient and her phenotypically healthy mother were estimated. The phenomenon of primary pigmentation occurred in the patient between 300 nm and 350 nm, at 310 nm being the shortest latency and the greatest intensity of pigmentation (irradiation time 30 sec., latency 20 and 16 days, resp.). The mother developed no pigmentation but an erythema

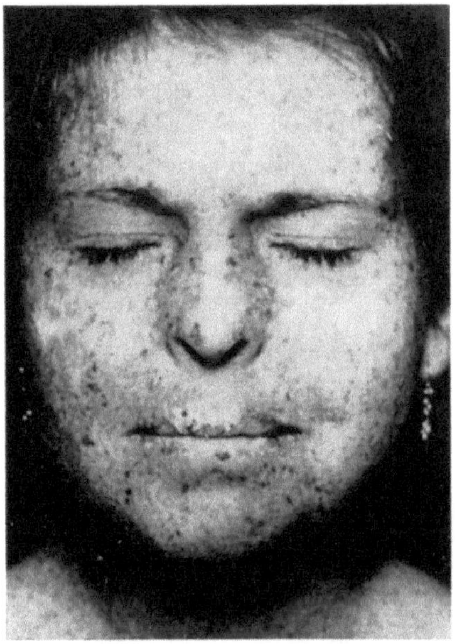

Fig. 3a

after 6 hours between 290 nm and 320 nm with its maximum at 300 nm and 310 nm and the longest duration between 290 nm and 310 nm (24 hours). With the fourfold radiation time of 2 minutes an erythema could be induced in our patient. It appeared after 6 hours between 290 nm and 350 nm, persisted for 12 days and shaded into long lasting pigmentation. In the same study the mother revealed an erythema after 6 hours between 260 nm and 330 nm with its maximum between 290 nm and 320 nm, which passed over into long lasting pigmentation after 72 hours, the maximum being between 300 nm and 320 nm.
The *3rd patient* (Leipzig) is a 29 years old female dispensary-clerk with no siblings and parents of no consanguinity.
The *skin alterations* corresponding to the first and second stages occurred soon in the first months of life. Already in the age of five the first squamous cell carcinoma of the face had to be removed. Meanwhile 100 neoplasias, mainly on the light-exposed skin were removed (Fig. 3a) and histologically examined, as listed in Table 1. Some tumours were

treated with x-rays or 5-Fluorouracil and are not listed, so that the total number of neoplasias is even higher. In 1972 the ablatio of the left breast was carried out on the suspicion of malignant melanoma which proved to be a necrotic adenoma.
In the present state of the disease freckle-like light to dark-brown pigmentations, depigmented spots, atrophies and teleangiectasias occur on the dry and pityriasiform-scaly skin of face (Fig. 3b, c), neck, trunk and limbs, mainly in the light-exposed parts of the body. The nose is rarefied in the distal portion. On the face and back one can find tumours which clinically are diagnosed as haemangiomas, actinic keratoses and basal cell epitheliomas (Fig. 3b, c).

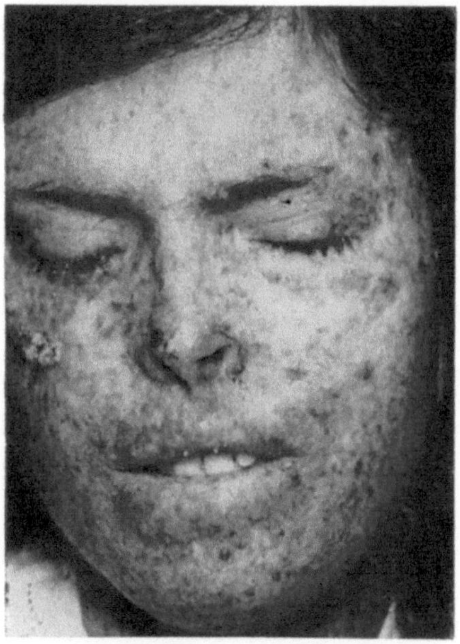

Fig. 3b

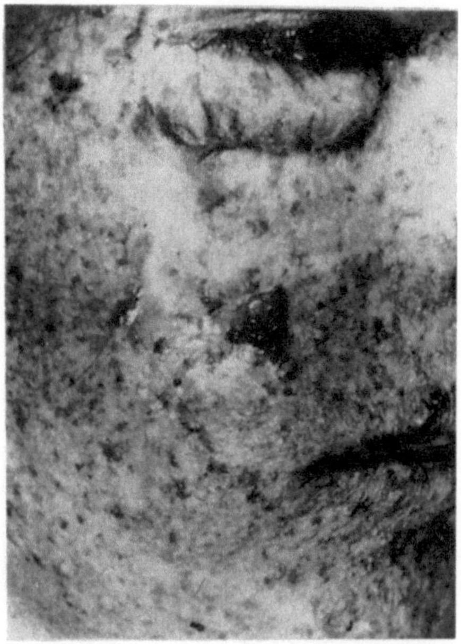

Fig. 3c

Fig. 3. a) 9-yaer-old girl (3rd patient) with numerous teleangiectasias, actinic keratoses and basaliomas. b) At the age of 26. Note the scarring, teleangiectasias and haemangiomas as well as the squamous cell carcinoma on the right cheek. c) Scarred poikilodermatous skin with haemangioma at the age of 29.

The *neurological* examination revealed no abnormalities; intelligence and degree of education are over the normal. The *ophthalmological* findings are: pronounced ectropium formation of the lower lids, on the left side being a condition after surgical removal of a squamous cell carcinoma, besides a strong conjunctival irritation. The right cornea shows parenchymatous opacity and superficial vascularization. The *chromosomal* analysis demonstrated a normal karyotype of 46 XX.
Specimens of four different regions from sun-unexposed, clinically tumour-free skin of this 29-years-old woman were investigated by electron microscopy: back, breast, abdomen, and thigh.

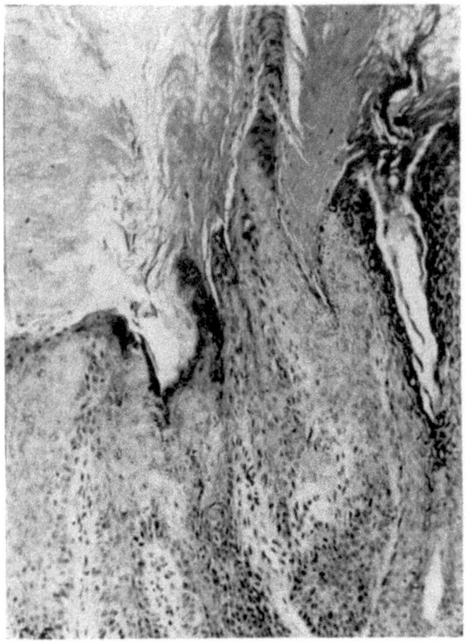

Fig. 4. Corum cutaneum on the basis of a papillomatous actinic keratosis.
haematoxylin-eosin, 200-fold
(microscop. magnific.)

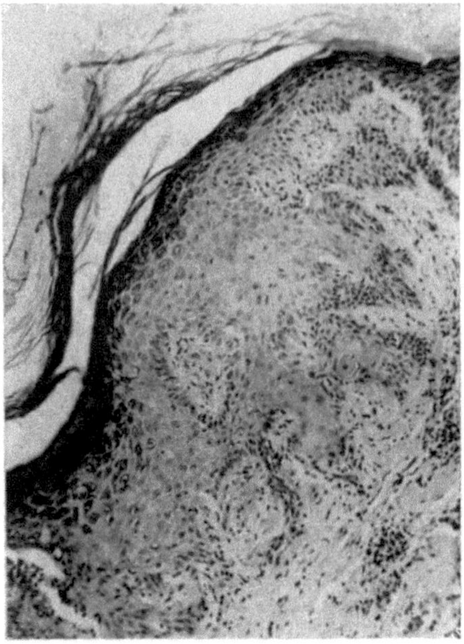

Fig. 5. Initiating squamous cell carcinoma on the basis of actinic keratosis.
haematoxylin-eosin, 200-fold
(microscop. magnific.)

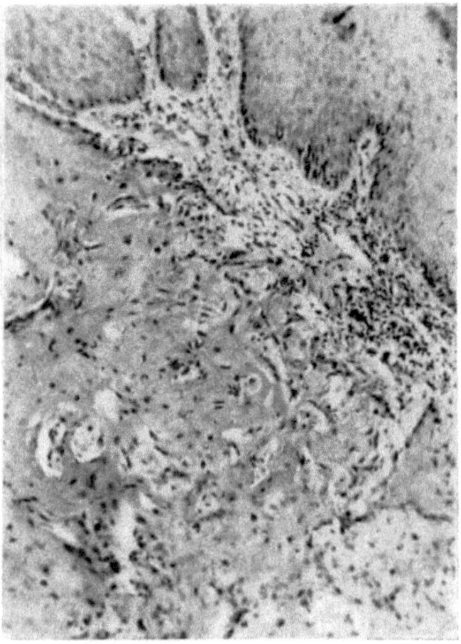

Fig. 6. Differentiated squamous cell carcinoma.
haematoxylin-eosin, 200-fold
(microscop. magnific.)

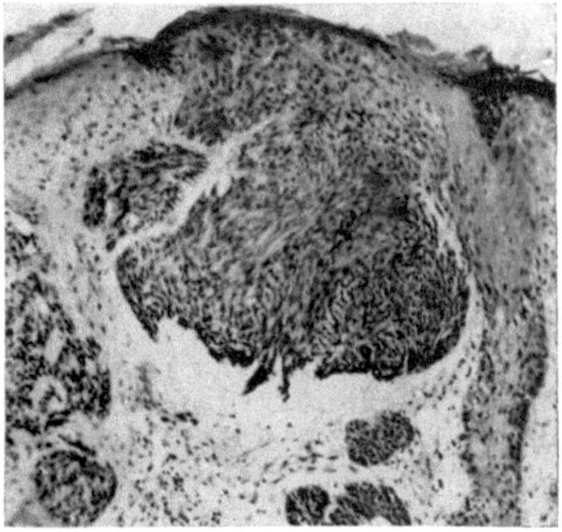

Fig. 7. Predominantly solid basalioma.
haematoxylin-eosin, 200-fold
(microscop. magnific.)

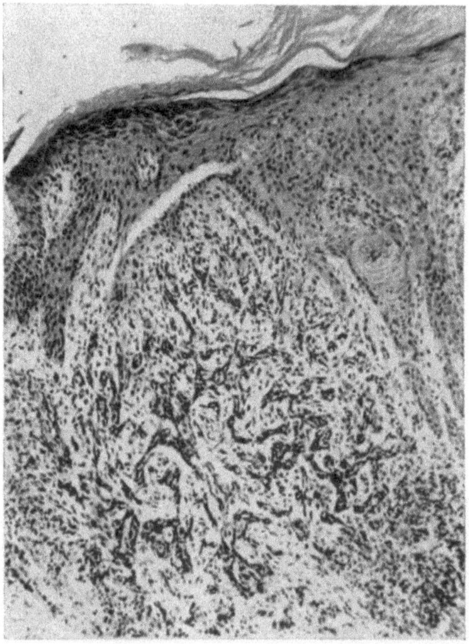

Fig. 8. Partly adenoid, partly scleroder-miform basalioma.
haematoxylin-eosin, 200-fold (microskop. magnific.)

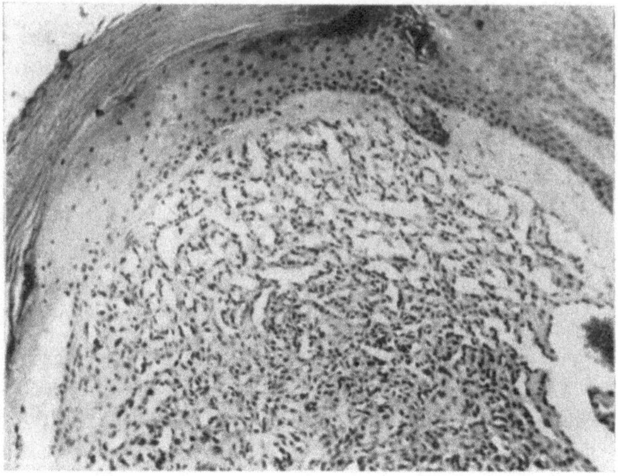

Fig. 9. Haemangioma
haematoxylin-eosin, 200-fold (microscop. magnific.)

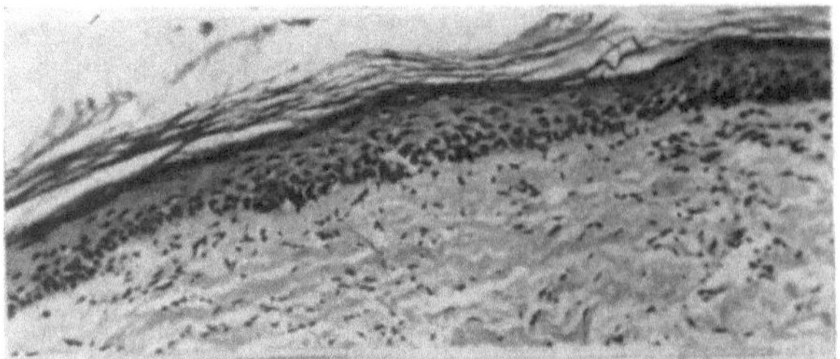

Fig. 10

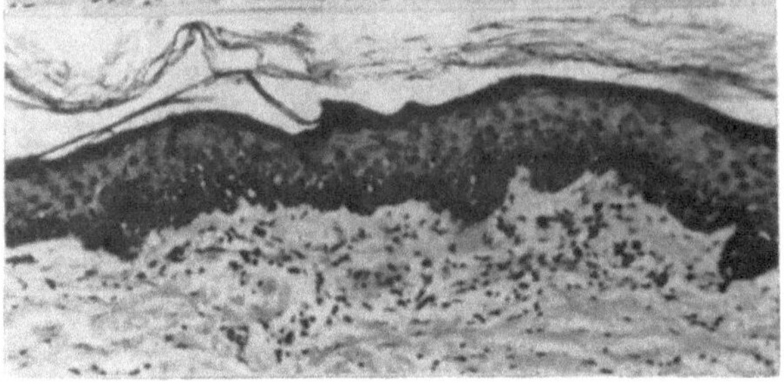

Fig. 11

Fig. 10. Atrophic epidermis with hyperpigmented basal cell layer and cicatrized corium. haematoxylin-eosin, 200-fold (microscop. magnific.)

Fig. 11. Lentigo maligna (Melanosis praeblastomatosa Dubreuilh) in the first stage. haematoxalin-eosin, 200-fold (microscop. magnific.)

Methods

Skin specimens were immediately sliced into 1 mm blocks, fixed in 3,2% glutaraldehyde in cacodylate buffer (0,1 N, pH 7,2) for 30 min, washed with the same buffer three times, postfixed in osmium tetroxide for 1 h (1% in cacodylate buffer: 0,1 N, pH 7,2), dehydrated through graded concentrations of ethanol and acetone, stained with 1% uranylacetate in 50% ethanol for 15—30 min immediately after 50% ethanol dehydration, embedded in Vestopal $W^{(R)}$, sectioned by the ultratome LKB, stained by Reynolds lead citrate solution and examined in the electron microscope at 60 kV. The pathological changes were also examined on semi-thin slices stained with toluidine blue.

Results

The number of cell layers of the epidermis is reduced. The stratum corneum of this atrophic epidermis is regularly arranged with A- and B-cells (no parakeratosis!), normal desmosome disks and cement membranes (Fig. 12). In places we find a large number of melanosomes in the horny cells, which were extruded. The stratum granulosum is reduced to 1 to 2 cell layers. The keratohyaline granules seem to be arranged more rarely and electron-lucent than normal (Fig. 12, 13), but enlarged in places. Tonofilaments are widely absent in this layer. The mitochondria are hydropically swollen, without cristae and occasionally ruptured. The cytoplasm is scarcely formed on account of the intracellular edema. The number of keratinosomes (membrane-coating granules, odland-bodies) is normal, the intercellular spaces and desmosomal connections are properly established (Fig. 13).

The keratinocytes of the spinous layer are very distinctly hydropically altered in places. Amorphous-granular substances as well as remnants of membrane-bordered organelles are localized in these giant structureless areas of the cytoplasm (Fig. 14, 15). Such clear edematous zones are situated partly around the nucleus, partly at the cell periphery. In these areas the tonofilaments are nearly absent, but partly also fragmented and elec-

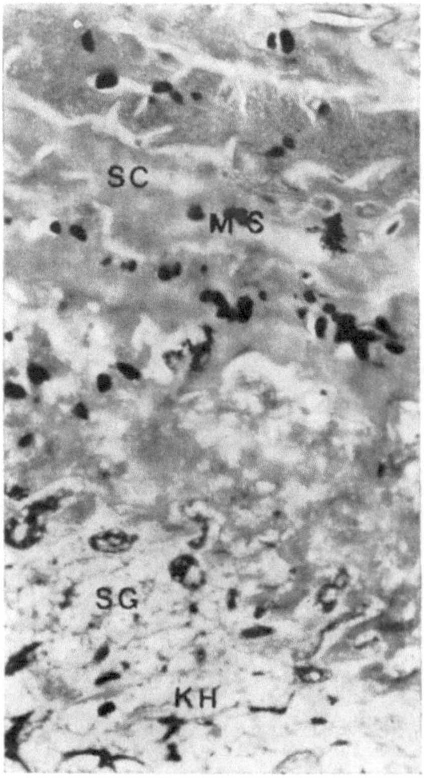

Fig. 12. Regular stratum corneum (SC) containing several melanosomes (MS). Stratum granulosum (SG) with small keratohyaline granules (KH).
8000-fold (microscop. magnific.)

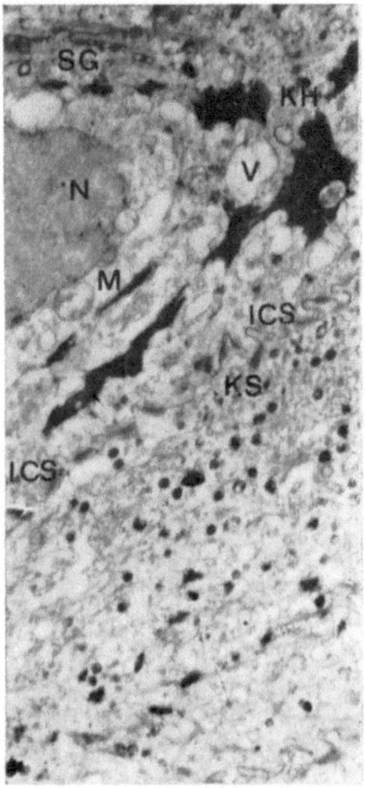

Fig. 13. Stratum granulosum (SG) with distinct keratohyaline granules (KH). Hydropically swollen mitochondria (M) and vacuoles (V) are situated perinuclearly. The intercellular space (ICS) and keratinosomes (KS) are normal. N = nucleus 8000-fold (microscop. magnific.)

tron-densely coarsened (Fig. 15). Ribosomes are scarcely to be seen. Sometimes the rough and smooth endoplasmic reticulum is enormously enlarged (Fig. 16). Here we find membrane-bordered vacuoles containing amorphous-granular substances (Fig. 14) as well as numerous hydropically degenerated mitochondria, among them numerous melanosome(complexes) (Fig. 17). Mostly the desmosomes are regularly formed, the intercellular space is relatively seldom enlarged, but in such cases with loss of the desmosomal contact and formation of microvilli. Often the nuclei of the keratinocytes are invaginated, hydropically swollen and contain up to three distinct nucleoli (Fig. 17) of different configuration.

The changes of the (prae)melanosomes we find in melanocytes, keratinocytes, horn cells and melanophages are remarkable. The number of melanocytes with extended dendrites is increased in the stratum basale and lower part of the stratum spinosum. The melanosome(complexes) are arranged partly in caps near the nucleus, partly they surround the whole nucleus (Fig. 18), partly they fill the whole cytoplasm of the cells. In cytoplasm they occur as single organelles or in membrane-bound complexes in polymorphous shape and size. Besides numerous praemelanosomes also ring structures, figures "en cocardes" and gigant melanosomes can occasionally be seen (Fig. 19a, b).

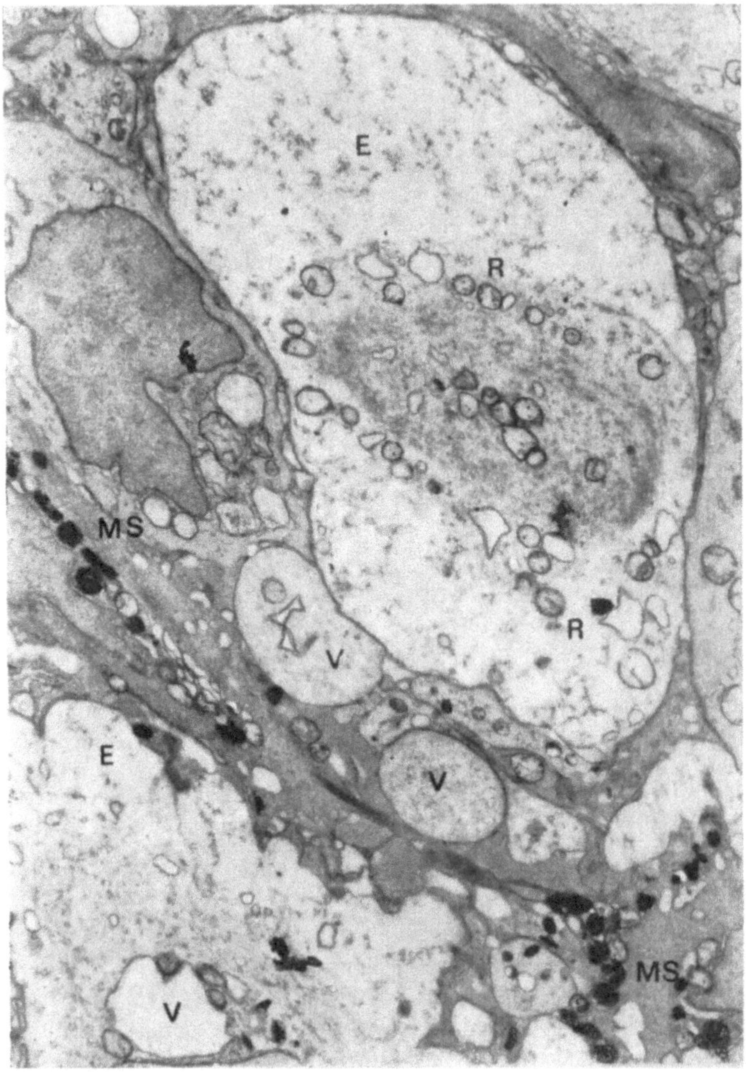

Fig. 14. Keratinocytes with massive intracellular edema (E) and remnants of organelles (R), as well as with melanosomes (MS) and vacuoles (V). Tonofilaments are nearly completely absent.
8000-fold (microscop. magnific.)

The junctional zone between epidermis and corium is mostly intact. The basement membrane shows sometimes a swollen and indistinct structure, but gaps, ruptures or reduplications could not be discovered. Especially the changes of the basal cells are evident. Large vacuoles, desintegration of cytoplasm, cytoplasmic edema with remnants of organelles (e.g. melanosomes) can be observed (Fig. 20, 21). Occasionally the endoplasmic reticulum is enormously enlarged, the mitochondria are distinctly swollen and without cristae (Fig. 20). Other basal cells exhibit condensed cytoplasm (Fig. 20), only scarce tonofibrils and perinuclear vacuoles.

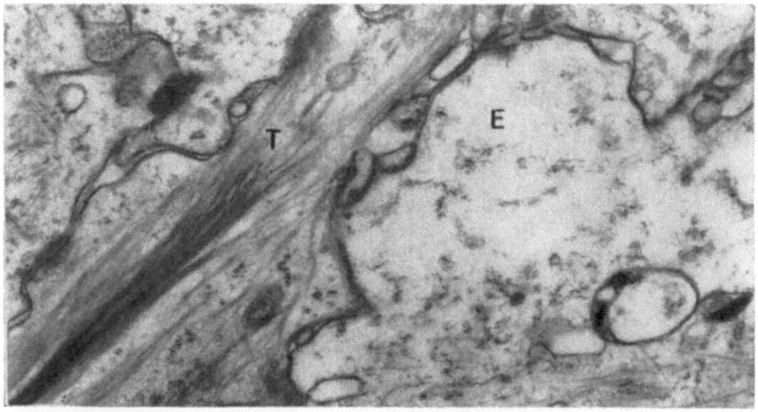

Fig. 15. Keratinocyte with intracytoplasmic edema (E). Beside is one with condensed tonofilaments (T).
16000-fold (microscop. magnific.)

Similar optically empty membrane-bordered vacuoles also occur in the upper corium near the basement membrane (Fig. 20, 21, 22). The elastic fibres show masses of dense grains and round holes in their matrix. The holes contain granular material, thin banded rings, round electron-dense bodies, several myelin figures and/or thin filaments with knobs. Elastic fibres were very scarce inside the holes. The collagen fibrils are normal with regard to the periodicity and diameter. Generally they exhibit minor alterations, although they are disintegrated by homogenous elastotic material and split into microfibrils, which are also produced by fibroblasts. The latter contain numerous organelles (swollen mitochondria, giant melanosomes, membrane-bordered vacuoles).
The endothelial cells of the blood vessels are distinctly swollen. Microvilli protrude into the lumen. Numerous pinocytotic vesicles, swollen mitochondria as well as small vacuoles can be observed. The perivascular basement membrane as well as the structure of the pericytes are without abnormalities.

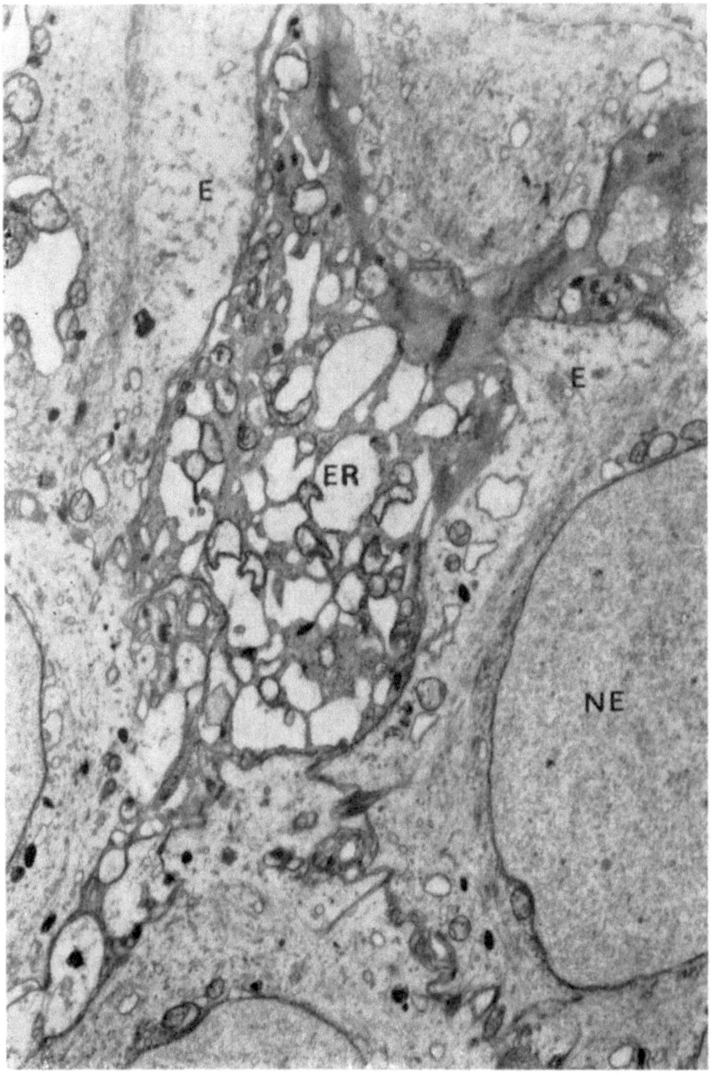

Fig. 16. Keratinocyte with enlarged endoplasmic reticulum (ER), other with peripheral intracellular edema (E) as well as intranuclear edema (NE). The intercellular space (ICS) seems to be normal.
8000-fold (microscop. magnific.)

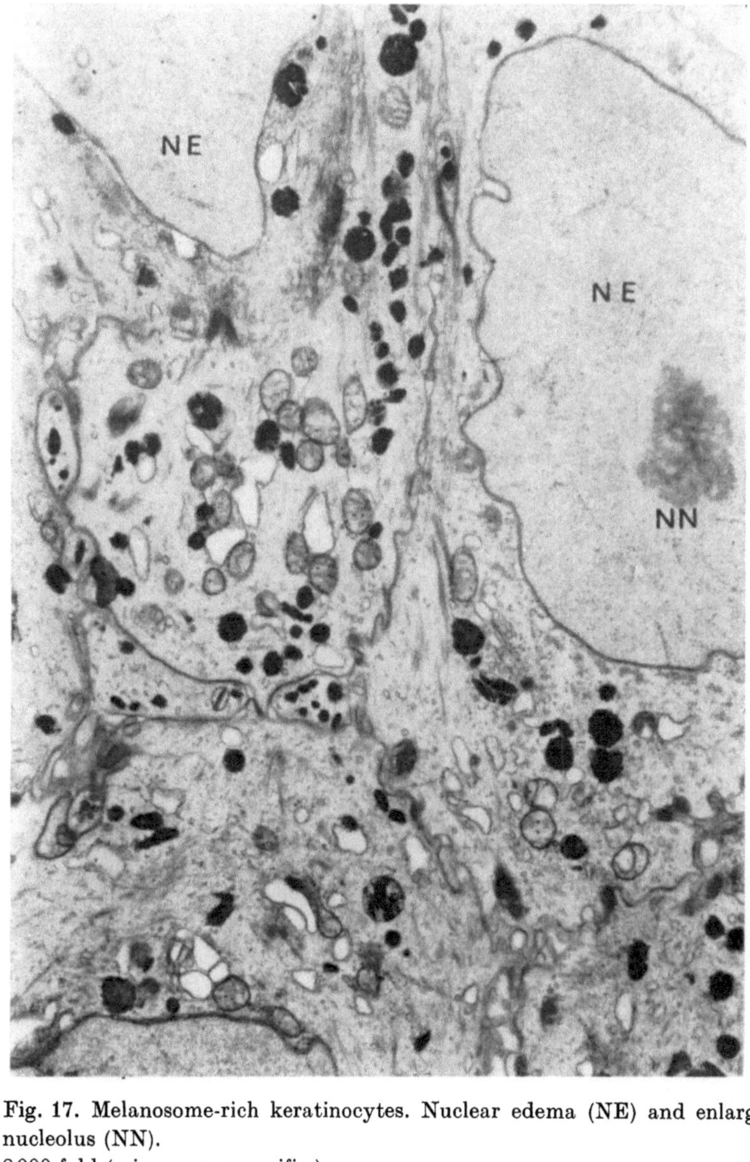

Fig. 17. Melanosome-rich keratinocytes. Nuclear edema (NE) and enlarged nucleolus (NN).
8000-fold (microscop. magnific.)

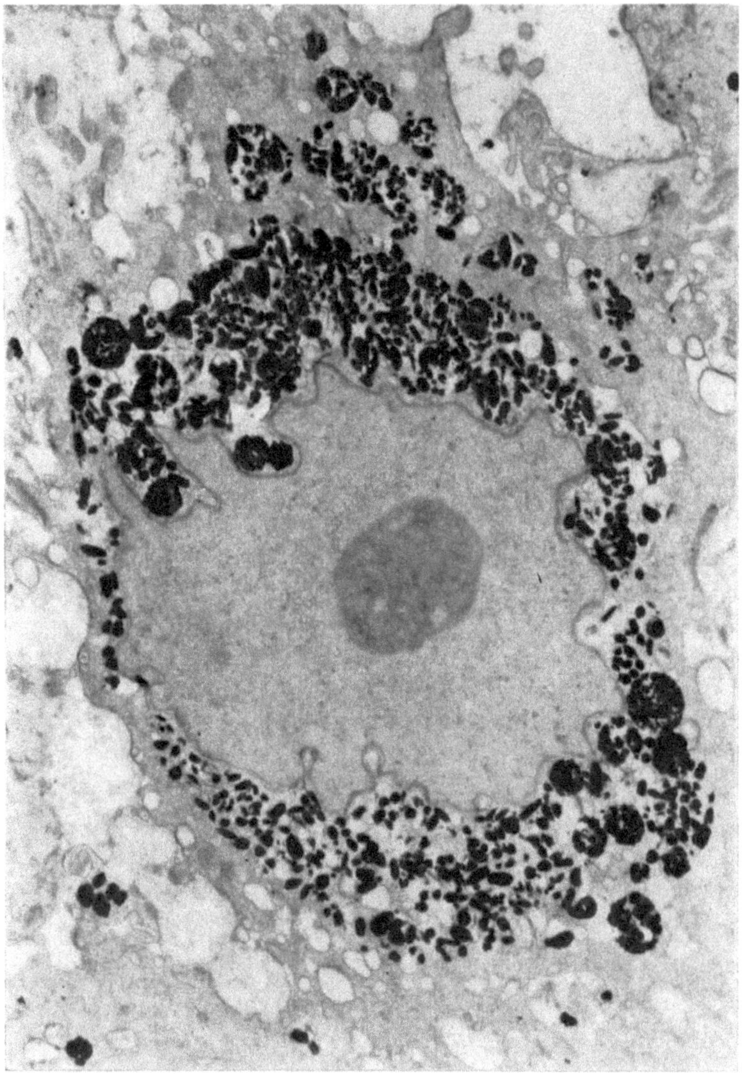

Fig. 18. Melanocyte totally filled with melanosomes.
8000-fold (microscop. magnific.)

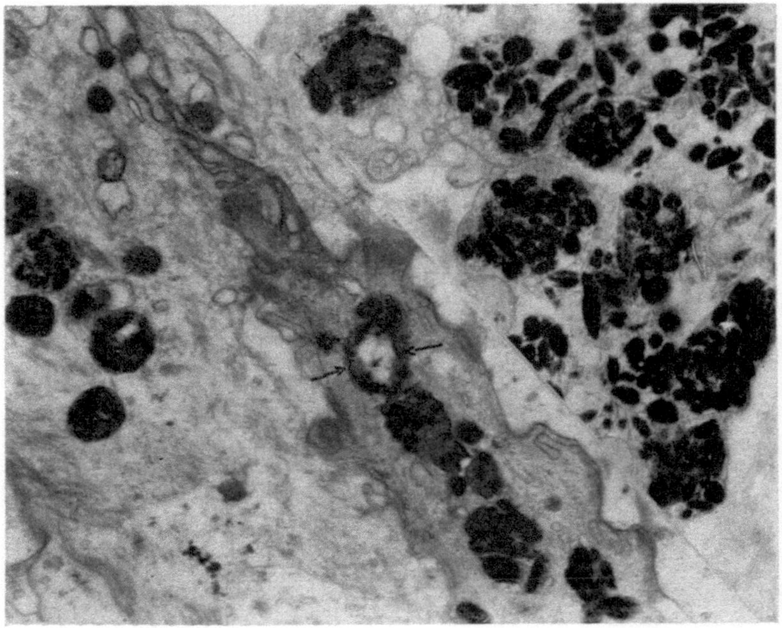

Fig. 19a and b. Prae(melanosomes) and -complexes (a, b), partly in ring configuration (arrow) in a dentritic process (a).
16000-fold (microscop. magnific.)

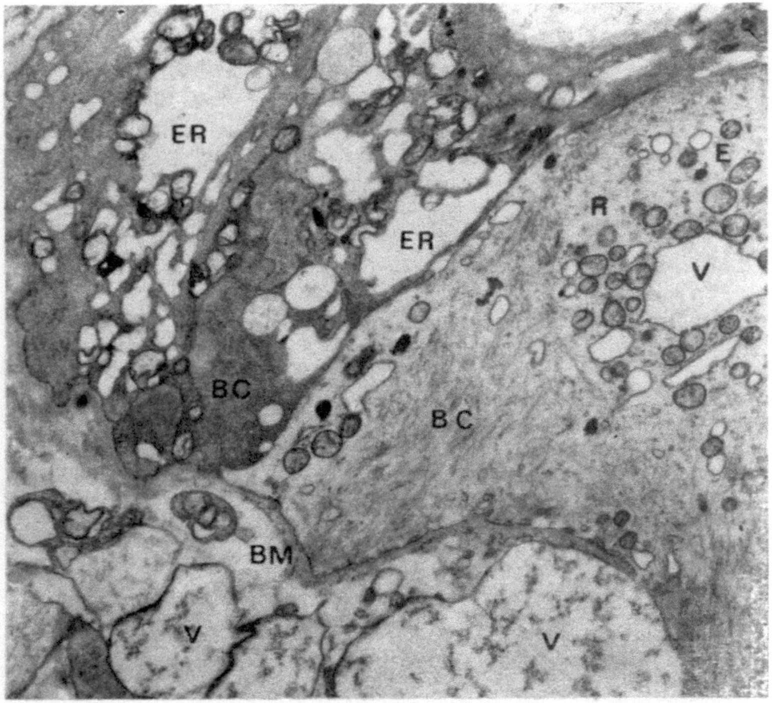

Fig. 20. Basal cells (BC) with intracellular edema (E), remnants of organelles (R), vacuoles (V) and enlarged endoplasmic reticulum (ER). The basal cell to the left shows condensed cytoplasm. Below the basement membrane (BM) large vacuoles are situated in the corium.
8000-fold (microscop. magnific.)

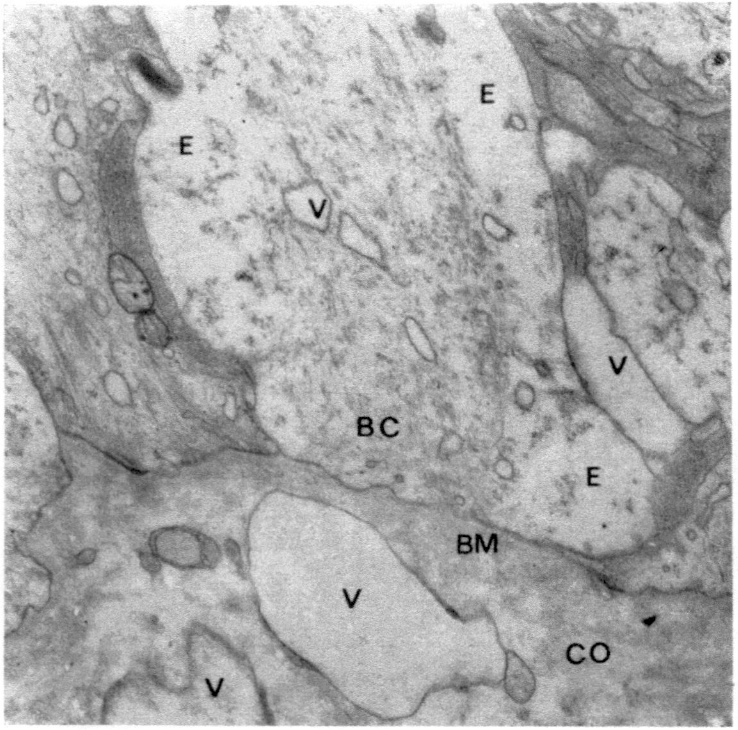

Fig. 21. Basal cell (BC) with vacuoles (V) and intracellular edema (E). Vacuoles also below the basement membrane (BM) in the corium (CO). 16000-fold (microscop. magnific.)

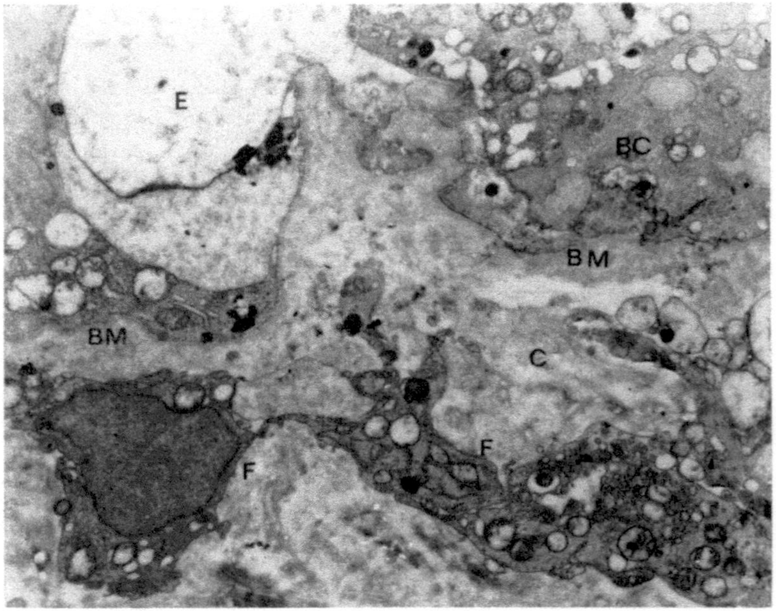

Fig. 22. Edematous (E) basal cell (BC) beside a condensed one. Fibroblast (F) with richness of organelles.
BM = basement membrane, C = collagen
8000-fold (microscop. magnific.)

Discussion

In all 3 patients described here the diagnosis X. p. is confirmed by the clinical course of this compulsory precancerosis with the development of numerous malignant tumours of the epidermal, mesenchymal and pigment forming system. Since the discovery of the fundamental disturbance of the dark repair of the DNA [5, 6, 35] the disease as a natural model of carcinogenesis has aroused the increasing interest of numerous oncologists, biochemists and radiation biologists.
Today X.p. can be classified into 4 phenotypically similar, but pathogenetically different, variants [20, 35]:

1. X.p. with defective dark repair [5, 6]
2. X.p. with defective postreplication repair (pigmented xerodermoid [16, 22]
3. X.p. with decreased content of photoreactivating enzyme (appr. 5% of the normal activity) [36, 37]
4. X.p. without any detectable DNS repair defects [7]

Which of these variants our patients belong to, is not yet clear. Probably the pigmented xerodermoid [16, 22] can clinically and histologically be excluded, because the skin shows distinctly atrophic changes. In all patients the illness started at early childhood. During the clinical course the stages of poikilodermia, precancerosis and malignancy (stages II—IV) could be observed.
No doubt the UV-light is the causative agent, because

(1) the skin changes in regions protected by clothes were less pronounced than in unprotected areas, especially in the face;
(2) the region of the bathing-shorts was nearly unaffected.

Having studied the cases of X.p. published in the literature no difference seems to be between normal and sick persons in regard to the dependence of the UV-erythema on energy (minimal erythema dosis), but often the erythema occurred with delay and persistence [8, 21]. Langhof et al. [21] emphazise that several of their X.p. patients did not develop any erythema after intensive natural or arteficial UV-exposure. In comparison to these findings our second patient showed only primary and persistent pigmentations, but her mother developed a temporary erythema under equal conditions. In this patient the action spectrum of the UV-light was shifted to longer waves concerning the pigmentation (patient: 330—350 μm, mother 300—320 μm) as well as the challenge of the erythema by the 4-fold irradiation dosis (patient 290—350 μm, mother 260—330 μm).
In two out of three patients the manifestation of tumour metastases could be prevented. In the Berlin patient the successful epithetic treatment of the nose defect should be emphazised. The nose had been removed because of a squamous cell cancer. But the exitus could not be prevented here. The two other patients are under permanent treatment, though an absolute light protection is not possible. The course of the disease demonstrates our therapeutic incapability always lagging behind the development of cancers. Besides the surgical and radiological treatment we also apply ointments containing cytostatics or light protectors (Colchicine, 5-Flourouracil, Contralum a.o.). Whether the regression of the cancer formation rate observed in our second patient since 1972 is due to the local treatment with 5-Flourouracil-containing ointment for

seven years or to a spontaneous regression rate, cannot be clearly distinguished. The photoprotective effect had been elaborated by several authors [10, 14, 17, 38, 42]. In our second patient the shifting from epidermal to mesenchymal tumours is remarkable, too. Since no pathogenetic treatment of this disease does exist so far, an important factor is the prophylaxis in form of a genetic consultation of affected families. Here the method of prenatal diagnosis of this genetic disorder described by REGAN et al. [33] should be applied.

Both the patients still living reached a relatively old age. Their discipline and understanding of the disease surely play a role. Both have qualified professions and do not show any neurological disturbances; this argues against the so-called de-Sanctis-Cacchione-Syndrome. The third patient is even married. But it should not be forgotten that the patients are socially isolated and in the worst psychological situation. The weak defense against infections partly observed in our patients were also described by others [32].

The electronmicroscopical investigation of the light-protected tumour-free skin of the third patient revealed

1. distinct changes of the epidermis, especially of the basal cells and lower layers of the spinous cells with diffuse intracellular edema, formation of vacuoles and defective differentiation of tonofilaments
2. activation of melanogenesis
3. vacuolization of the upper corium and changes like "sensile" elastosis.

ad 1: changes of the keratinocytes and basal cells:

These findings remind of light-induced changes with the skin carefully light-protected by clothes being likely to acquire a latent damage everywhere. In comparison to the results of NAGY et al. [25] who divided the postirradiation changes into two phases we observed the mainly exsudative phenomena of the first phase: distinct intra- and less intercellular edema, vacuolization of cytoplasm [25, 27, 28] and swelling of the nucleus of the basal cells and keratinocytes. The degenerative processes of the second phase, however, were not marked to such an obvious degree because condensation of the cytoplasm and retraction of the tonofilaments and of the desmosomes were rather discrete, but the pycnosis of the nucleus was completely missing.

The origin and function of vacuoles are unknown [1.]. Possibly they arise from large invaginations of the plasma membrane. But some cells contained only membrane-free spaces in form of diffusely decreased cytoplasmic density and no membrane-lined vacuoles. [2.] Therefore the formation of vacuoles might be a secondary event. Vacuolar membranes could then fuse with plasma membranes and permit discharge of vacuolar contents into the extracellular space. [3.] Thirdly the vacuoles might derive from enlargement of membrane enclosed organelles, e.g. GOLGI-vesicles [27].

We found only slight signs of initiating dyskeratosis (vacuolization, decrease of the number of desmosomes, nucleolar enlargement, perinuclear edema) in contrast with the dyskeratosis observed after UV-irradiation [25] or in precancerous stages of UV-exposed skin (squamous and dyskeratotic lesions) in X.p. [3]. In such stages qualitatively and quantitatively enhanced alterations could be registered: mitoses, irregularities of the nucleus with invaginations and inclusions, especially hypertrophy and structural changes of the nucleoli which is to be interpreted as a substrate of precancerous stages, but not as diagnostic criteria of cell malignancy [3]. The nucleolar enlargement seems to be manifestation of increased metabolic activity of these cells. Wier et al. [40] found electron dense clumps in shrunken, vacuolated and disorganized nuclei, which were related to earliest morphological changes occurring after UV-light irradiation in human epidermis and may be signs of decreased RNA and protein synthesis. Neither typical edematous dyskeratotic "sunburn cells" [30] nor structures resembling anchoring fibrils and the basal lamina and located within the grossly dilated rough endoplasmic reticulum of some basal and suprabasal keratinocytes [39] could be identified.

Contrary to Rasheed et al. [31], Caputo and Califano [3] we could not observe distinct enlargements of the intercellular spaces with rupture of the cytoplasmatic membranes and release of cell contents (e. g. melanosomes) into the intercellular space as well as the occurrence of microvilli-like protrusions of the cytoplasm of the keratinocytes. The desmosomes were intact as a rule. The tonofilaments are rarefied, occasionally fragmented and electrondensely coarsened.

In comparison to acute UV-injuries neither the decrease of the number of keratinosomes [41] nor "irregular dense bodies" [27] could be found. The latter were interpreted as complexes of glycolipids or glycoproteins. The keratinosomes have several features in common with lysosomes (acid phosphatase activity, origin in the Golgi-area, lipid content [43]). Because of their lamellated structure, their existence only in malpighian and granular cells as well as their secretion into the extracellular space they are not identical with lysosomes [29, 41]. Although lysosomal lysis accompanies UV-reaction of the epidermis—by the way, not as an initial event [13] — we could not find any signs of lysosomal involvement in X.p. Thus it is very doubtful whether the keratinosomes are the reason for the "spotty" appearance of cell changes [15] or not.

The keratohyaline granules in the lowermost cells were partly enlarged and relatively electron-lucent [31]. Only two layers of stratum granulosum could be observed. Contrary to UV-induced changes the stratum corneum was not parakeratotic and showed normal structure with desmosome disks, cement membranes, complete keratinization and keratin pattern, although the orthokeratotic zone included a number of well-preserved melanin granules.

ad 2: activation of the melanogenesis:

The findings registered in melanocytes were also described in X.p. by other authors [11, 31]: polymorphous praemelanosomes and melanosomes of varying shape, size and internal structure, partly with less developed matrix, their arrangement "en cocarde", formation of giant pigment granules, asynchrony in melanization, passage of melanosomes to keratinocytes, containing them as single organelles or membrane-bordered complexes, their loss through the corneal cells, and phagocytosis by melanophages in the corium. But we could not observe any dentritic processes of melanocytes passing through the basement membrane. All these findings are signs of an accelerated formation of (prae)melanosomes and its complexes as observed also in lentigo senilis [2] or in malignant melanoma, both possible complications of X.p.

The enormous melanosome complexes in keratinocytes may represent an effort on the part of the cells of the epidermis to protect themselves against the deleterious effects of UV-light. The considerable number of praemelanosomes in the keratinocytes could reflect an increased output of pigment by melanocytes in response to increased demand on the part of the keratinocyte and subsequently insufficient time for full maturation within the melanocyte [11]. Futhermore the question arises whether disturbances in melanin degradation play any role, because the single melanosomes are to be found in all layers of the epidermis including the stratum corneum. The lack of phagolysosomes as well as of LANGERHANS-cells containing melanosomes support this assumption. Quantitative electron microscopic study following two weeks of daily UV irradiation revealed an increase in melanocyte number and an absence of LANGERHANS-cells suggesting some form of relationship between both the cell types [44, 45]. These findings were similar to ours, but contrary to these of GUERRIER et al. [11], who observed elevated numbers of LANGERHANS-cells bearing large quantities of melanin.

Finally CESARINI et al. [4] investigated hypopigmented macules of sun-unexposed skin and found a vitiligo-like situation. In melanocytes and LANGERHANS-cells melanin granules were either rare or absent. The white spots therefore were not protected by pigment against UV-irradiation. Apart from the genetic enzymatic DNA-repair defect the authors conclude from these findings a genetic melanocytic abnormality leading to an elevated sensitivity to UV-irradiation as an additional pathogenetic factor.

ad 3: vacuolization and "senile" elastosis:

According to BRAUN-FALCO [1] as well as DANIELSEN and KOBAYASHI [9] the elastotic fibrils consisted of elastotic matrix, microfibrils and electron-dense inclusions. The alterations of the elastic and collagen fibres in the upper corium may be interpreted as the consequence of the elevated UV-damage [31]. The origin of the elastotic material is still unclear, because the histogenetic interpretation of such amorphous material is especially problematic [1, 24, 26]. Partially the microfibrils observed in elastotic material may derive from splitting collagen fibrils, partially they may be produced by fibroblasts [1]. We relate the approximately normal structure of the fibroblasts with signs of active metabolism to the small depth of penetration of the UV-light into the skin tissue, since the defects of dark repair of fibroblasts were predominantly demonstrated in vitro, but not in vivo.

Summary:

Report on 3 female patients (12†, 22 and 29 years old) suffering from xeroderma pigmentosum. The clinical pictures and courses of the disease are presented during the erythematous, poikilodermatous, precancerous and neoplastic stages. The patients developed a great number of epidermal (actinic keratosis, basalioma, squamous cell carcinoma, keratoakanthoma), mesenchymal (haemangioma, granuloma pyogenicum, (angio)fibroma, histiocytoma) and pigment forming tumours (lentigo senilis, lentigo maligna) in early childhood. Surgical, radiological as well as local treatment with cytostatic ointments were carried out. The light protection is insufficient in regard to the prophylaxis of the formation of new tumours, because an etiological treatment of the DNA repair defect is not possible and an effective undangerous light protection drug is not known.

The elctron microscopical investigations of the sun-unexposed tumour-free skin covered by clothes revealed

1. distinct changes of the keratinocytes and basal cells: intracellular edema of high degree, formation of vacuoles, alteration of mitochondria, rarefication of tonofilaments, swelling of the nucleus, but seldom also condensation of the cytoplasm.

2. a pronounced polymorphism and a definite increase in the number of (prae)melanosomes
3. Vacuolization of the upper corium and formation of microfibrils and elastotic material, changes which are comparable with the so-called elastosis.

The structure of fibroblasts is widely normal, possibly because of the little penetration depth of the UV-light.
The changes are interpreted as and compared with UV-induced damages. The increased and accelerated melanin synthesis may be explained as a compensatory protective phenomen against UV-irradiation, which also may lead to a malignant transformation like in lentigo maligna or malignant melanoma. The "senile" elastosis and vacuolization in the upper corium also seems to be the consequence of UV-irradiation and defect repair mechanism. In our specimens of tumour-free skin neither cytoplasmic nor nuclear alterations were found, which could be regarded as diagnostic signs of cell malignancy.

References

[1] Braun-Falco, O.: Die Morphogenese der senil-aktinischen Elastose; Eine elektronenmikroskopische Untersuchung. Arch. klin. exp. Derm. **235**, 138–160 (1969)

[2] Braun-Falco, O., Schoefinius, H. H.: Lentigo senilis — Übersicht und eigene Untersuchungen; Hautarzt **22**, 277–282 (1971)

[3] Caputo, R., Califano, A.: Ultrastructural changes in the epidermis of Xeroderma pigmentosum lesions in various stages of development; Arch. Derm. Forsch. **241**, 364–373 (1971)

[4] Cesarini, J. P., Bioulac, P., Moreno, G., Prunieras, M.: Hypopigmented macules of sun-unexposed skin in Xeroderma pigmentosum. An electron microscopic study; J. Cutaneous Pathol. **2**, 128–139 (1975)

[5] Cleaver, J. E.: Defective repair replication of DNA in Xeroderma pigmentosum; Nature (Lond.) **218**, 652–656 (1968)

[6] Cleaver, J. E.: DNA damage and repair in light sensitive human skin disease; J. Invest. Derm. **54**, 181–195 (1970)

[7] Cleaver, J. E.: Xeroderma pigmentosum: Variants with normal DNA repair and normal sensitivity to ultraviolet light. J. Invest. Derm. **58**, 124–128 (1972)

[8] Cripps, D. J., Ramsay, C. A., Ruch, D. M.: Xeroderma pigmentosum: Abnormal monochromatic action spectrum and autoradiographic studies; J. Invest. Derm. **56**, 281–286 (1971)

[9] Danielsen, L., Kobayashi, T.: Degeneration of dermal elastic fibres in relation to age and light-exposure; Preliminary report on electron microscopic studies; Acta Dermatovener. **52**, 1–10 (1972)

[10] Diem, E.: 5-Fluoro-Uracilbehandlung aktinischer Keratosen bei Xeroderma pigmentosum; Z. Haut-Geschl. Krkh. **48**, 29 (1973)

[11] Guerrier, C. J., Lutzner, M. A., Devico, V., Prunieras, M.: An electron microscopical study of the skin in 18 cases of Xeroderma pigmentosum; Dermatologica **146**, 211–221 (1973)

[12] Hoede, K.: Xeroderma pigmentosum: in Dermatologie und Venerologie; Bd. IV, herausgeg. H. A. Gottron und W. Schönfeld, S. 48–53, G. Thieme: Stuttgart 1960

[13] Hönigsmann, H., Wolff, K., Konrad, K.: Epidermal lysosomes and ultraviolet light; J. Invest. Derm. **63**, 337–342 (1974)

[14] Ippen, H.: Untersuchungen zur Lichtphysiologie der Haut. I. Erythemschutz durch externe Anwendung von 5-Fluorouracil; Arch. klin. exp. Derm. **234**, 204–212 (1969)

[15] Johnson, B. E., Daniels, F.: Lysosomes and the reaction of skin to ultraviolet radiation; J. Invest. Derm. **53**, 85 (1969)

16] Jung, E. G., Schnyder, U. W.: Xeroderma pigmentosum und pigmentiertes Xerodermoid; Schweiz. med. Wschr. **100**, 1718—1726 (1970)

[17] Kahn, G., Curry, M. C., Dustin, R.: UV protective effects of 5-Fluorouracil and Thymidine; Dermatologica **147**, 97—103 (1973)

[18] Klaschka, F.: Xeroderma pigmentosum und Lungenmetastasen; Z. Haut-Geschl. Krkh. **31**, 297—309 (1961)

[19] Korn-Heydt, G. E.: Xeroderma pigmentosum: in Handbuch der Haut- und Geschlechtskrankh.; Erg. werk, herausgeg. J. Jadassohn Bd. VII, S. 608—616, Springer: Berlin—Heidelberg—New York 1966

[20] Kraemer, K. H., Coon, H. G., Petinga, R. A., Barrett, S. F., Rahe, A. E., Robbins, J. H.: Genetic heterogeneity in Xeroderma pigmentosum: Complementation groups and their relationship to DNA repair rates; Proc. nat. Acad. Sci **72**, 59—63 (1975)

[21] Langhof, H., Rietschel, L., Feuerstein, M.: Xeroderma pigmentosum; Arch. klin. exp. Derm. **216**, 391—401 (1963)

[22] Lehmann, A. R., Kirk-Bell, S., Arlett, C. F., Paterson, M. C., Lohmann, P. H. M., de Weerd-Kastelein, E. A., Bootsma, D.: Xeroderma pigmentosum cells with normal levels of excision repair have a defect in DNA synthesis after UV-irradiation; Proc. nat. Acad. Sci **72**, 219—223 (1975)

[23] Meffert, H.: Kasuistischer Beitrag zum Xeroderma pigmentosum; Pädiatrie und Grenzgebiete **13**, 177—182 (1974)

[24] Mitchell, R. E.: Chronic solar dermatosis: a light and electron microscopic study of the dermis; J. Invest. Derm. **48**, 203—220 (1967)

[25] Nagy, G., Wiskemann, A., Schneider, G.: Feinstrukturelle Veränderungen der Epidermis nach UV-Licht-Bestrahlung; Strahlentherapie **138**, 627—639 (1969)

[26] Niebauer, G., Stockinger, L.: Über die senile Elastosis. Histochemische und elektronenmikroskopische Untersuchungen; Arch. klin. exp. Derm. **221**, 122—143 (1965)

[27] Nix, T. E. jr., Nordquist, R. E., Scott, J. R., Everett, M. A.: Ultrastructural changes induced by ultraviolet light in human epidermis: basal and spinous layers; J. Invest. Derm. **45**, 52 (1965)

[28] Nix, T. E.: Ultraviolet induced changes in epidermis. In Zelickson, A. S. (ed.) Ultrastructure of normal and abnormal epidermis; p 304—319, Lea & Febinger Publ., Philadelphia 1967

[29] Odland, G. F., Reed, T. H.: Epidermis. In: Ultrastructure of normal and abnormal skin (Ed. by A. S. Zelickson), p. 54—75, Lea & Febinger, Philadelphia 1967

[30] Olson, R. L., Gaylor, J., Everett, M. A.: Ultraviolet-induced individual cell keratinization; J. Cutan. Pathol. **1**, 120—125 (1974)

[31] Rasheed, A., El-Hefnawi, H., Nagy, G., Wiskemann, A.: Elektronenmikroskopische Untersuchungen bei Xeroderma pigmentosum; Arch. klin. exp. Derm. **234**, 321—344 (1969)

[32] Reed, W. B., Sanding, B., Sugarman, G., Cleaver, J. E., Melnyk, J.: Xeroderma pigmentosum. Clinical and laboratory investigation of its basic defect; J. amer. med. Ass. **207**, 2073—2079 (1969)

[33] Regan, J. D., Setlow, R. B., Kaback, M. M., Howell, R. R., Klein, E., Burgess, G.: Xeroderma pigmentosum: A rapid sensitive method for prenatal diagnosis; Science (Wash.) **174**, 150 (1971)

[34] Schnyder, U. W.: Xeroderma pigmentosum: in Doerr, W., G. Seifert, E. Uehlinger: Spezielle pathologische Anatomie — Haut und Anhangsgebilde; S. 242, Springer: Berlin—Heidelberg—New York 1973

[35] Sönnichsen, N., Meffert, H.: Störung der DNS-Reparatur beim Xeroderma pigmentosum; Derm. Mschr. **159**, 849—859 (1973)

[36] Sutherland, B. M., Oliver, R.: Low levels of photoreactivating enzyme in Xeroderma pigmentosum variants; Nature (Lond.) 257, 132—134 (1975)

[37] SUTHERLAND, B. M., RICE, W., WAGNER, E. K.: Xeroderma pigmentosum cells contain low levels of photoreactivating enzyme; Proc nat. Acad. Sci. **72**, 103—107 (1975)

[38] TRONNIER, H.: Weitere Untersuchungen zur Lichtschutzwirkung von 5-Fluoruracil; Strahlentherapie **141**, 748—751 (1971)

[39] TSUJI, T.: Electron microscopic studies of xeroderma pigmentosum: unusual changes in the keratinocyte; Brit. J. Derm. **91**, 657—666 (1974)

[40] WIER, K. A., FUKUYAMA, K., EPSTEIN, W. L.: Nuclear changes during ultraviolet light-induced depression of ribonucleic acid and protein synthesis in human epidermis; Labor. Invest. **25**, 451—456 (1971)

[41] WILGRAM, G. F., KIDD, R. L., KRAWCZYK, W. S., COLE, P. L.: Sunburn effect on keratinosomes; A report with special note on ultraviolet-induced dyskeratosis; Arch. Derm. **101**, 505 bis 520 (1970)

[42] WISKEMANN, A.: Pharmakologischer Lichtschutz durch Bausteine der Nukleinsäuren im Tierversuch; Strahlentherapie **141**, 752—755 (1971)

[43] WOLFF, K., HOLUBAR, K.: Keratinosomen als epidermale Lysosomen; Arch. klin. exp. Derm. **231**, 1 (1967)

[44] ZELICKSON, A. S.: Melanocyte, melanin granule and LANGERHANS-cell; in: Ultrastructure of normal and abnormal skin, ZELICKSON, A. S. ed., p 163—182, Lea & Febinger Philadelphia 1967

[45] ZELICKSON, A. S., MOTTAZ, J.: The effect of sunlight on human epidermis; A quantitative electron microscopic study of dentritic cells; Arch. Derm. **101**, 312—316 (1970)

Effects of UV-Light on DNA Synthesis in Photodermatoses.

I. Horkay, M. D., L. Varga, M. D., P. Tamási, M. D., S. Gundy, M. D. and E. Nagy, M. D.

[Dept. of Dermatology, University Medical School of Debrecen, 4012, and "Frederic Joliot- Curie" National Research Institute for Radiobiology and Radiohygiene, Budapest 22, Hungary]

Ultraviolet irradiation of healthy human epidermal cells results in changes in DNA synthesis which can be demonstrated by autoradiographs using tritiated thymidine as the radioactive tracer to label nuclei [7, 9]. One of these changes occurs immediately and lasts several hours after irradiation and represents unscheduled or repair DNA synthesis. This phenomenon is characterized by uniform sparse 3—15 grains per cell labelling of the majority of epidermal nuclei of the basal, malpighian and granular layers that means incorporation of monomeric thymidine to replace pyrimidine dimers formed in UV-damaged DNA molecules ("excision repair"). The other effect of UV-light is on the semiconservative DNA synthesis autoradiographically reflected in quantitative changes of heavily labelled — more than 15 grains per cell — basal and epibasal cells that make DNA in the *S*-phase of the mitotic cycle. 3—5 hours after UV-irradiation an early depression of these cells occurs followed by a recovery within 24 hours resulting in a 3 to 6-fold increase in their number.

It is mainly xeroderma pigmentosum that UV-light induced changes in DNA synthesis have been studied so far. In this rare genodermatosis with light sensitivity associated with high incidence of cutaneous malignancies a severe defect in excision repair due to enzymatic disturbance can be detected in the epidermal cells, cultured corial fibroblasts and peripheral lymphocytes [2, 4, 8, 12]. On the other hand only few observations concern these UV-light induced DNA changes in other dermatoses influenced by light (e.g. keratosis solaris: 14, lupus erythematosus: 1, 3, 11).

The aim of our work was to study the repair of UV-light induced DNA damage and changes in the semiconservative DNA synthesis in the epidermis of patients with some lightdermatoses caused primarily by sunlight and of patients suffering from xeroderma pigmentosum. As for lightdermatoses, as far as we know, no similar investigations have been conducted so far.

Persons investigated: 8 patients with polymorphic light eruption (PLE), a clinical entity characterized by pleomorphic skin changes confined primarily to sun-exposed sites and provoked by sunburn range. This skin disorder is considered to be a manifestation of photoallergy mostly of delayed type [6]; 7 patients with porphyria cutanea tarda and erythropoietic protoporphyria caused by a hereditary or an acquired enzymatic disturbance in the porphyrin metabolism and provoked phototoxically by long-wave UV-light; 1 patient with xeroderma pigmentosum (XP) and 6 control persons without any light sensitivity.

Investigations were performed in summer using the skin of patients with florid clinical symptoms. The minimal erythema dose (MED) was first established by means of a 250 watt germicidal lamp (type Medicor Q) at 24 hours for the patients and the controls on the symptomfree skin of the upper back of the trunk. Then the skin was irradiated with three times the MED on one occasion in all subjects and another skin area with five times the MED daily for four consecutive days. This is what EPSTEIN describes as the repeated phototest for reproduction of the original skin symptoms [5]. Biopsies were secured as follows: from the skin irradiated with three times the MED 2 and 48 hours after irradiation, from the repeated phototest sites on the fifth day. In addition biopsies were taken from unirradiated control sites as well as from the florid skin eruptions of the patients with lightdermatoses. All the biopsy speciemens were immediately placed in Parker TC 199 medium containing 15 microCi/ml tritiated thymidine with a specific activity of 5 Ci/mM. After incubation at 37 °C for 4 hours skin biopsies were removed, washed twice with isotope free culture medium, fixed in formalin; then paraffin sections were prepared and cut at 3 micron thickness. Then the slides were coated with Ilford G5 emulsion and after 7 days' exposure developed and stained with haematoxylin and eosin. Incorporation of the labelled thymidine was measured autoradiographically. The nuclei of more than 2000 cells were counted in each section. Two types of nuclear labelling were observed: heavily labelling/more than 15 grains per cell/representing basal and epibasal cells in *S*-phase and sparse labelling (3—15 grains per cell) representing cells of the basal, malpighian and granular layers in repair incorporation. Results are expressed in the percentage of the labelled nuclei. The statistical analysis was carried out by the T test.

Results

As regards the semiconservative DNA synthesis demonstrated autoradiographically by heavily labelled nuclei of the basal and epibasal cells (Fig. 1.) in the biopsy specimens of persons investigated, our findings are shown in figures. The percentage of these cells

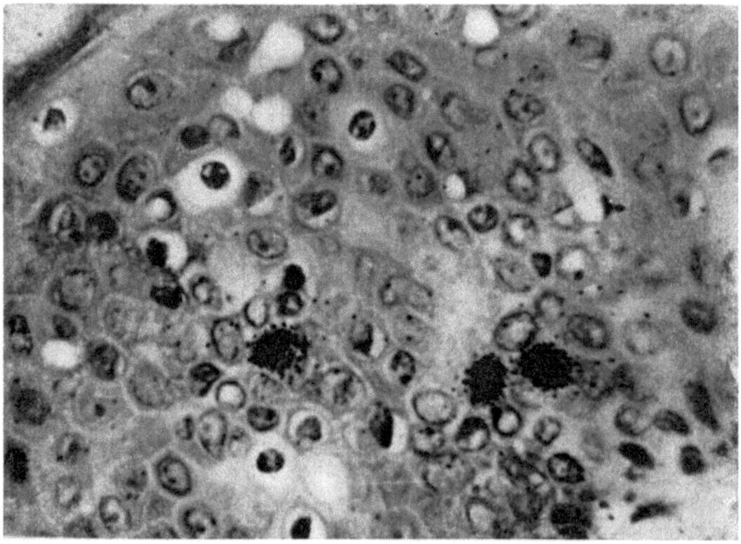

Fig. 1. Autoradiograph of the normal unirradiated skin of the upper back of the trunk. Man aged 45. The incorporation of the tritiated thymidine into the germinative basal cells during the *S*-phase is demonstrated by the heavily nuclear labelling. [×400]

in the unirradiated and symptomfree skin of the controls and patients with lightdermatosis does not differ significantly; its value ranges from 1.74 to 3.07 in agreement with the literary data [4, 10, 13]. In biopsy specimens taken from the skin irradiated with three times the MED 2 hours after UV-irradiation a slight but statistically not significant early depression in the percentage of the heavily labelled nuclei can be observed in patients and controls. 48 hours after irradiation a highly significant increase (p is less than 0.01) occurs in all four groups investigated. It is especially remarkable in the skin obtained from patients with polymorphic light eruption (PLE) and in that of the controls whereas in cases with cutaneous porphyrias (CP) it is of far less degree (Fig. 2).

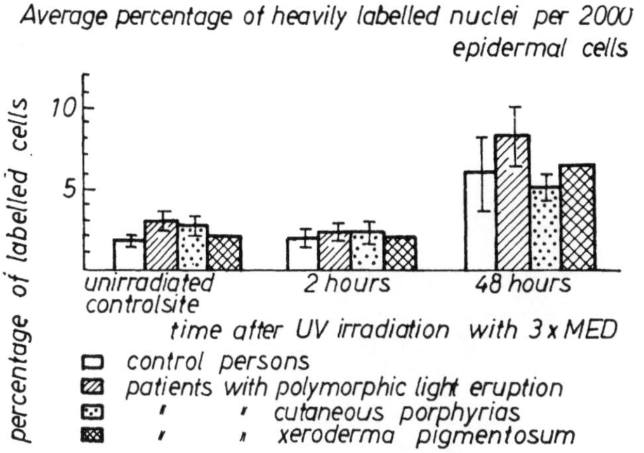

Fig. 2

The percentage of the heavily labelled nuclei in the biopsy specimens obtained from the clinical eruptions and the symptomfree control skin site of the patients can be seen in Fig. 3. In each group of subjects the difference is statistically insignificant but as for averages in PLE it is remarkable even if not significant because of the great standard deviation.

Finally on the skin irradiated daily with five times the MED that is on the site of the repeated phototest, the original skin symptoms of the patients with PLE were repro-

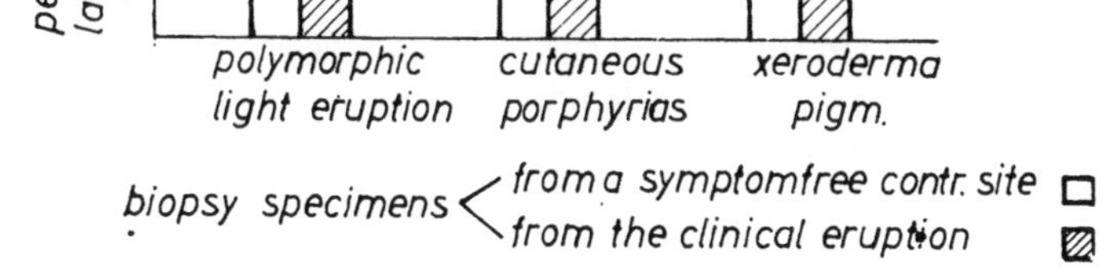

Fig. 3

duced similar to EPSTEIN's-findings [5] whereas in cases with CP and in those of the controls a usual erythematous sunburn reaction was observed. In the biopsy specimens obtained from these sites the number of heavily labelled cells was higher than that of the unirradiated control site. The difference is considerable in each group investigated.
Our further findings concern the unscheduled or repair DNA synthesis demonstrated autoradiographically by sparsely labelled epidermal nuclei (Fig. 4). As it is shown in Fig. 5 the average percentage of these cells 2 hours after UV-irradiation with three times the MED does not differ significantly in cases with PLE and CP. Repair incorporation

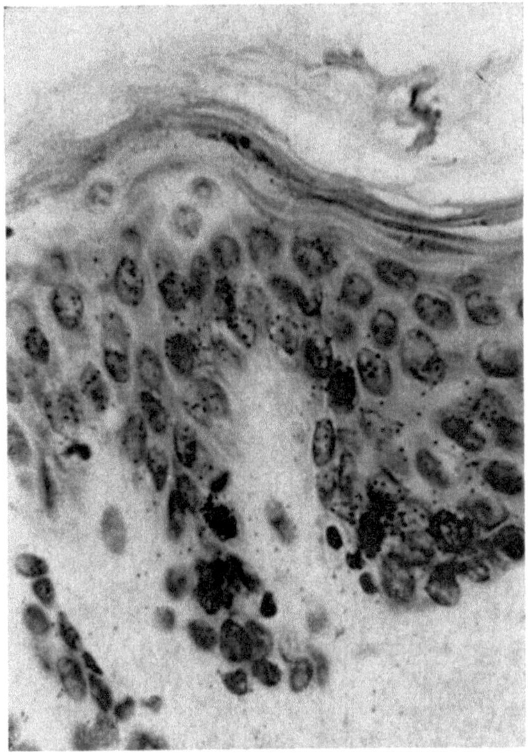

Fig. 4. Unscheduled DNA synthesis in the epidermal cells 2 hours after UV-irradiation is demonstrated by the sparse labelling in the majority of the nuclei. PLE patient aged 35. [×400]

can be detected in 70—80% of the cells. In contrast xeroderma pigmentosum (XP) is characterized by a very low repair capacity in agreement with the literary findings [4, 8]. The intensity of the repair synthesis is demonstrated in Fig. 6. The average grain-count per cell in PLE is similar to that of the controls whereas it is significantly lower in cases with CP and especially in XP. On the basis of the findings concerning the DNA synthesis after UV-irradiation our case is to be considered a variant of XP in which the semiconservative and above all the repair synthesis is significantly reduced but can be demonstrated. — 48 hours after irradiation no thymidine incorporation indicating repair synthesis could be detected in the biopsy specimens of any groups investigated. It means

that the repair process has been completed by this time as it is confirmed by the literary data [7]. It can explain one of our further findings, namely, no repair incorporation can be observed in the specimens obtained from the repeated phototest site or from the florid skin eruptions 24 hours after irradiation.
Conclusions are to be drawn very cautiously because of the great individual differences in the DNA synthesis detected in our study. However our present results suggest some

Average percentage of sparsely labelled nuclei per 2000 epidermal cells 2 hours after UV-irradiation with 3 x MED

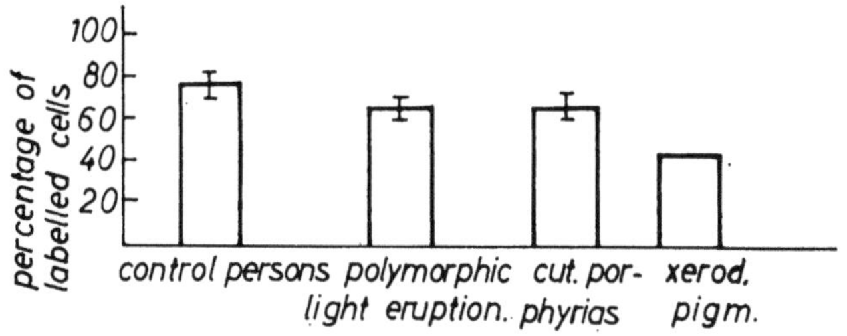

Fig. 5

Average grain-count per cell in repair synthesis 2 hours after UV-irradiation with 3 x MED

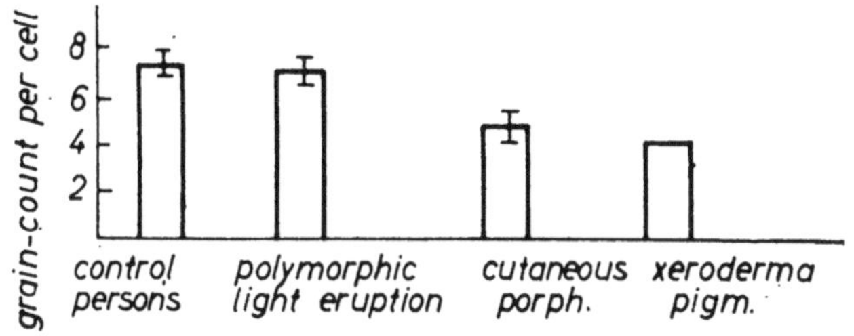

Fig. 6

alterations in both the semiconservative and the repair DNA synthesis in the epidermis of patients with lightdermatosis. Further studies will help in a better understanding of the pathomechanism not sufficiently cleared up in these skin disorders. Investigations in PLE seem to be especially worth-while since the nature of the proantigen presumably in the epidermis has not been identified so far [6]. Studying UV-light induced changes in the DNA synthesis can yield further informations.

References

[1] Altmann, H., Eberl, R.: Wiss. Ztschr. Friedrich-Schiller-Univ. Jena, Math.-Nat. R., **20**, 477 (1971)
[2] Cleaver, J. E.: Nature **218**, 652 (1968)
[3] Cleaver, J. E.: J. Invest. Derm. **54**, 181 (1970)
[4] Cripps, D. J., Ramsay, C. A., Ruch, D. M.: J. Invest. Derm. **56**, 281 (1971)

[5] Epstein, J. H.: Arch. Derm. **85**, 502 (1962)
[6] Epstein, J. H.: Ann. All. **24**, 397 (1966)
[7] Epstein, W. L., Fukuyama, K., Epstein, J. H.: Arch. Derm. **100**, 84 (1969)
[8] Epstein, J. H. Fukuyama, K., Reed, W. B., Epstein, W. L.: Science **168**, 1477 (1970)
[9] Epstein, W. L., Fukuyama, K., Epstein, J. H.: Fed. Proc. **30**, 1766 (1971)
[10] Fukuyama, K., Nakanura, T., Bernstein, I. A.: J. Invest. Derm. **44**, 29 (1965)
[11] Horkay, I., Nagy, E., Tamási, P., Szabó, M., Csongor, J.: Studia Biophys. **50**, 1 (1975)
[12] Jung, E. G.: Arch. Derm. Forsch. **241**, 33 (1971)
[13] Lachapelle, J. M., Gillman, T.: Br. J. Derm. **81**, 603 (1969)
[14] Lambert, B., Ringborg, U., Swanbeck, G.: VII. Internat. Congr. on Photobiology, Rome, 1976. P 160.

Defective Repair of γ-Irradiated DNA in a Case of Xeroderma Pigmentosum

V. M. Mikhelson

Institute of Cytology of the Academy of Sciencés of the USSR Leningrad

Great progress has been achieved in the study of cell repair mechanisms, especially of postradiation repair, as a result of the impressive success in bacterial biochemistry. Similar works on mammalian cells has begun relatively recently.
There are two main approaches, which are generally used in order to study DNA repair mechanisms. The first one is the repression of separate steps of repair by specific inhibitors. This approach requires a search for such inhibitors. The second way is the studying of repair processes in mutants, defective in different steps of repair. This approach requires a search for such mutants.
We tried both these approaches (Haykazyan et al., 1973), but the most interesting results, I believe, were obtained on mutants with defects in repair.
The study of molecular defects in human hereditary diseases is important not only for elucidation of human DNA repair mechanisms, but also for understanding of the biochemical fundamentals of carcinogenesis, for cell and organism senility theories, for clearing up of the relations between DNA repair and cell survival.
Human mutants with DNA repair defects were found only during the last decade. In 1972 we found a mutant with defective repair of γ-injured DNA (Mikhelson, Haykazyan, 1972).

Place of mutant, we found, among other mutations with repair defects

The first mutation of this kind was the classic form of Xeroderma pigmentosum (XP) — a rare human hereditary disease. The repair processes in XP cells were first examined by Cleaver (1968). Since then the number of known mutants with repair defects has been growing continually. All the first mutants discovered were defective in repair of UV-damaged DNA. We have found the first mutation which leads to deficiency in γ-damaged DNA repair — a form of XP, named XP II. Later some other human mutants with defects in repair of γ-lesions were found — progeria, ataxia-telangiectasia. All known human mutants, defective in DNA repair, are recessive diseases. A rough estimation of these genes frequency would be of the order of 1:100 — 1:350 (Passarge, 1972).
The enzymatic defect for some of these diseases has been ascertained exactly, for other — has been suggested with certain degree of probability, for third — is absolutely unknown.
These diseases can be divided in three groups:

I group unites the diseases with the nosological name Xeroderma pigmentosum. The main clinical symptoms of all the XP forms are the following: high sensitivity of skin to UV-rays, pigmentary changes in skin (freckles), sometimes mental retardation and sharply increased frequency of malignization. It is possible to distinguish 4 forms of XP:

1) Classic form of XP (or form I) with defective excision rerair of UV-damaged DNA (Cleaver, 1968; 1969) and normal repair of γ-lesions (Kleijer et al., 1970; Mikhelson et al., 1974). Within this form there are 5 genetically different types — groups of complementation (De Weerd-Kastelein et al., 1972; 1977). In all 5 groups the defective enzyme is UV-endonuclease (Tanaka et al., 1975).
2) Form XP II, that we found, with defect not only in excision repair of UV-damaged DNA, but also in restitution of γ-induced breaks of DNA (Mikhelson, Haykazyan, 1972).
3) "Variant" form of XP, described in 1971—1973 (Burk et al., 1971; Cleaver, 1972) with normal excision repair of UV-lesions and normal repair of γ-breaks, but is defective in postreplicative repair of UV-irradiated DNA (Lehmann et al., 1975).
4) So-called "Pigmented xerodermoid", described by Jung (1970; 1971; 1973). It is characterized by a normal level of repair of both UV and γ-lesions in DNA, but has delayed replicative DNA synthesis.

II group — diseases, united as "Chromosomal breakage syndrome" or "Syndrome of spontaneous chromosomal instability". Some authors (Passarge, 1972) include XP also into this group, but generally it consists of 3 diseases, characterized by the following common symptoms: sharply increased frequency of both spontaneous and induced chromosome aberrations; pigmentation disorder and other skin injuries, especially telangiectasias; stunted growth and somethimes mental retardation; reduced lifetime; susceptibility to leukemias and other malignizations.

1) Fanconi's-anemia is a hereditary hypoplastic pancytopenia (Fanconi, 1927). Poon et al. (1974) found the deficiency of excision of UV-induced dimers in Fanconi's-anemia cells. The incision of dimers, however, was normal. So, it may be a defect of UV-exonuclease. Defective excision of DNA cross-links in Fanconi's-anemia cells was described (Fujivara, 1975).
2) Ataxia-telangiectasia or Louis-Bar syndrome is a neurovascular disease (Louis-Bar, 1941) with cerebellar ataxia and oculo-cutaneous symmetrical telangiectasis. Recently it has been reported (Paterson et al., 1977) that ataxia cells are markedly deficient in excision repair of γ-modified base residues, but appear to be ordinary in their response to UV radiation. So, this disease is a γ-sensitive analogue of classic XP.
3) Bloom's-syndrome (Bloom, 1954). Till now no disorders in DNA repair have been found in its cells, though all the ways of repair within reach of estimation have been investigated (Cleaver, 1970, etc.). Thus, numbering of Bloom's-syndrom among the diseases with defective DNA repair is based on the suggestion that excessive chromosome breaking must surely result from disorder in some mechanisms of DNA repair. Strictly speaking, it is not necessary.

III group — diseases of premature senility. Because of extreme rarity of such diseases, its inheritance is unknown. Usually two forms of progeria are distinguished:

1) Hutchinson-Gilford progeria (Hutchinson, 1886; Gilford, 1904) begins in early childhood by symptoms of aging — grey hair, alopecia, atherosclerosis, wrinkled skin, etc. Patients usually die at age before 20 with all manifestations of deep senility. It is

known (GOLDSTEIN, 1969; 1971) that progeria skin fibroblasts in culture undergo a limited number of generations and are somewhat difficult to maintain: under ideal conditions progeria cells could not be carried beyond the 14-th generation, meanwhile, normal fibroblasts — up to 50—60 generations. EPSTEIN et al. (1973) reported that fibroblasts from progeria patient failed to rejoin single-strand breaks in DNA, induced by γ-irradiation (the same picture as in the cells of XP II — Fig. 2). Though REGAN and SETLOW (1974) supported these results only partially, in subsequent works of EPSTEIN and co-workers (EPSTEIN et al., 1974; LITTLE et al., 1974; BROWN et al., 1976) and of other authors (CLEAVER et al., 1975; ARLETT, 1977) defect of DNA breaks repair in γ-irradiated progeria cells was shown.

2) WERNER's-syndrome is a form of precocious senility with later begining and not so severe manifestations as in HUTCHINSON-GILFORD progeria. This form has not been studied well biochemically.

Besides these there are some other hereditary diseases with defects in DNA or chromosome repair: COCKAINE's-syndrome (WADE et al., 1977), sclerodermia (EMERIT et al., 1971; 1974), DOWN's-syndrome (LAMBERT et al., 1977).
Not only XP, but all other diseases with defective DNA repair are genetically heterogeneous (SCHROEDER et al., 1976; PATERSON et al., 1977). So, existence of different forms of XP is not surprising.

Clinical manifestations in XP II patient

The case of XP with γ-hypersensitivity of cells was found in 1972. Actually, the first data were published earlier (MIKHELSON, 1970; 1971), but at that time nothing was known about heterogeneity of XP, and it did not enter our heads to consider this case as a special form of XP.
Our patient has typical manifestations of XP. She is 22 years old now, Russian. She comes from very little village in Novgoro ddistrict, far fromr ailway — so it is possible to expect inbreeding. It is impossible to say exactly, if her parents are related, but it cannot be ruled out. Her mother and elder sister are phenotypically healthy (we have examined them). The father of the patient, according to her words, has some sort of pigmentation disorder. The patient has been suffering from the early childhood after UV-treatment of the whole body (we do not know the reason of that treatment). All the skin, except palms and soles, is covered with freckles and dry (Fig. 1). Atrophic skin and pigmentation spots disfigure the face. The patient has cloudings in the corneas and is nearly completely blind. She has a certain, but not very distinct mental retardation. There are no tumours till late — an unusual phenomenon for age of patient and severity of the disease.
This case is the only XP patient described with defect in γ-injured DNA repair. But in medical literature such cases were mentioned. In the twenties several authors (HEINER, 1925; MARTENSTEIN, BOBOWITCH, 1926) described patients with XP to be hypersensitive to X- and α-rays in the in vivo experiments. During subsequent years such in vivo experiments have not been carried out because of its danger, which became clear. But later SHANIN (1952; 1969) noticed that radiation therapy of skin cancer, developed in XP, sometimes led to acute attack of the basic disease. It can be supposed that those patients with increased sensitivity to ionizing radiation suffered from XP in form II.

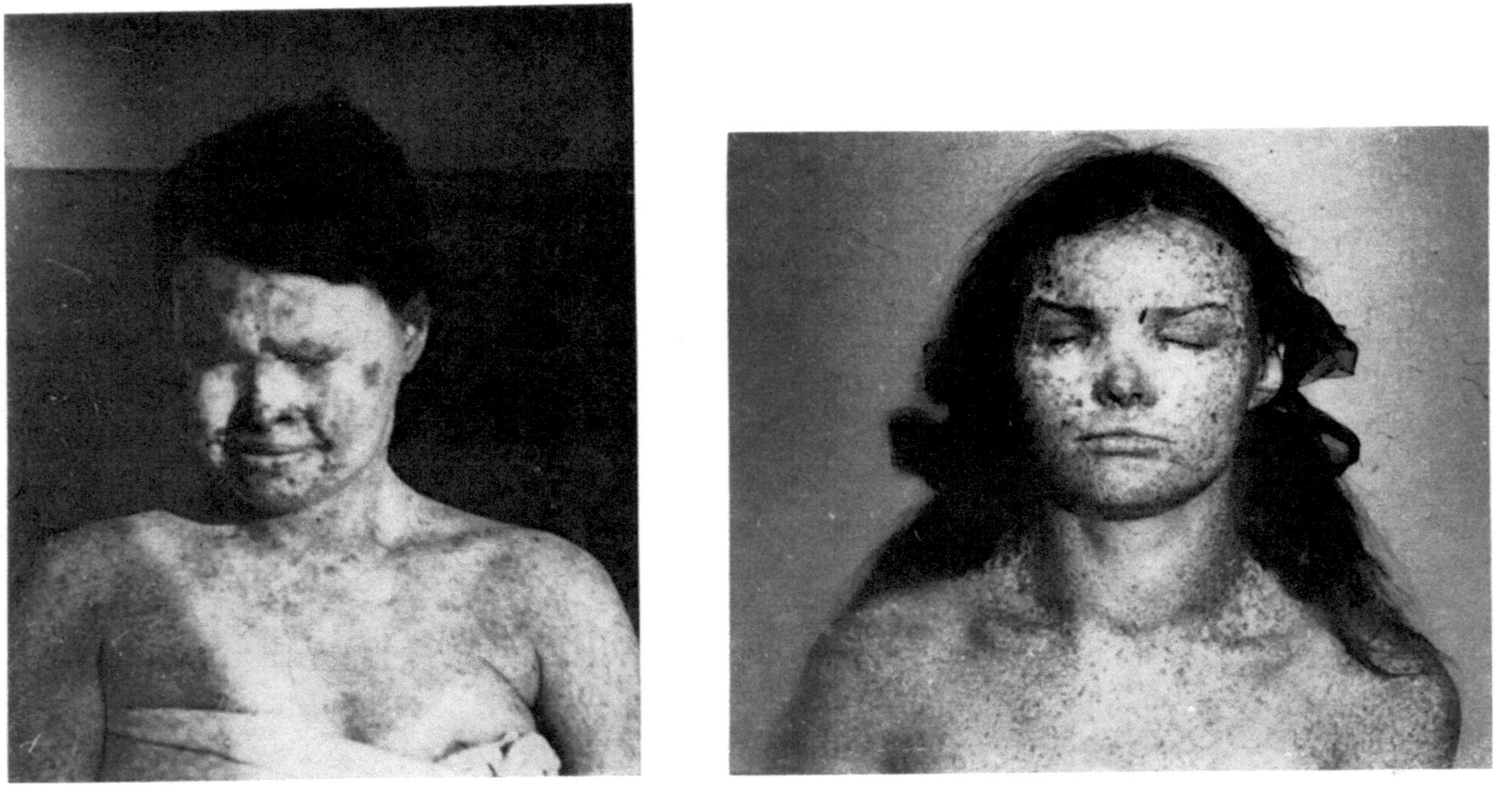

Fig. 1. Two XP patients we study:

a — XP1LE, classic form (Chuvash woman, 25 years old, died 1975 through lip cancer),

b — XP2LE, form II (Russian woman, 20 years old).

DNA repair defects in XP II cells

Nearby all biochemical and cytological studies of XP II were carried out on lymphocytes of peripheral blood. Only recently we began to work on cultured skin fibroblasts of XP patients. We use cells of our XP II patient (we name these cells XP2LE) and four non-related patients with classic form of XP (XP1LE, XP3LE, XP4LE and XP1MO), cells of XP II patient's mother — XPH2LE, and normal donor cells.
In experiments studying the rejoining of single-strand DNA breaks, lymphocytes were grown in a medium containing ^{3}H-thymidine and irradiated with 10, 20 or 30 krad of γ-rays at the temperature of melting ice. Irradiated cultures were frozen at-70° either immediately after irradiation, or in 30 or more minutes of incubation at 37°. After melting, lymphocytes were selected, lyzed and then were put on the top of an isokinetic alkaline sucrose gradient (5—26,5%) and centrifuged at 24000 revolutions per minute

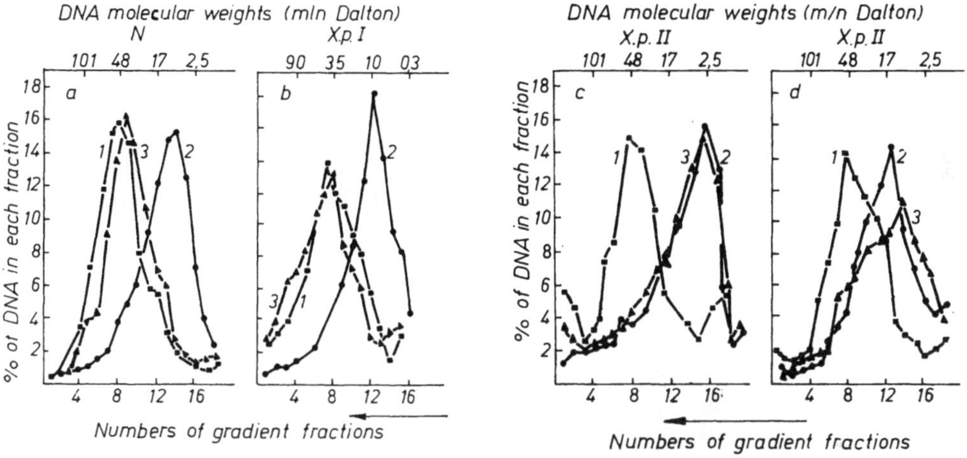

Fig. 2. Rejoining of single-strand DNA breaks in normal (a), classic XP (b) and XP II (c, d) lymphocytes, irradiated by 20 krad of γ-rays.
1 — without irradiation, 2 — immediately after irradiation, 3 — in 60 min (a, b, c) or 120 min (d) incubation after irradiation.

for 4 hours in SW-25-1 swinging bucket rotor of a Spinco centrifuge. Fractionation of the gradient and radioactivity assay were performed and weight-average molecular weights were calculated.
In Fig. 2 one can see that irradiation at 20 krad lowers the mol. weight of DNA in normal cells from 40—50 mlns Dalton to nearly 5 mlns (a). The same picture is for the cells of classic XP (XP1LE) and XP II (XP2LE). Postradiation incubation of normal and classic XP cells during 60 min. leads to increasing of DNA mol weight up to the initial position, which indicates rejoining of majority of single-strand breakes, induced by radiation (a, b). On the contrary, in the irradiated cells of XP II neither 60-min (c), nor more prolonged incubation (2 hours in Fig. d) leads to increase in molecular weight. So, the single-strand breaks in DNA of XP II lymphocytes fail to rejoin.
It is known that the cells of classic XP are deficient in UV-endonuclease enzyme, which performs the incision step in excision repair of UV-irradiated DNA (Tanaka et al., 1975). In the case of XP II the defect cannot be caused by UV-endonuclease, first of

all because this enzyme is not necessary for rejoining of γ-induced single-strand DNA breaks (see Fig. 2b). We suggest that cells XP2LE are deficient in some other enzyme — it might be either DNA-polymerase, or polynucleotid-ligase, because both of them are necessary for UV- and γ-damaged DNA repair. There are publications about insufficiency of DNA-polymerase in the cells of some XP patients (Müller et al., 1973). We cannot also rule out that XP2LE defect is due to double mutation. Indeed, several cases of combination of XP with other hereditary diseases in one patient were described (Goht, Cleaver, 1975).

The study of unscheduled DNA synthesis level in XP2LE cells gives us some more elucidation of the problem, what enzyme is defective in XP II. We have studied unscheduled DNA synthesis in lymphocytes after UV- and γ-irradiation. Lymphocytes were incubated in a medium without PHA — so, practically no cells were in the S-phase of cellular cycle. Thus, all the DNA synthesis registered was unscheduled, induced by irradiation.

The lymphocyte cultures were exposed to UV-doses of 5, 10, 20 and 30 J/m^2, then 2-hr impulse labeling was performed immediately and every 2 hrs during 24 hrs after irradiation. The cells were then fixed, the preparations were covered by photosensitive emulsion and exposed for 8 weeks at +4°. After developing and staining, the number of grains over the nucleus was counted. Nuclei with number of grains overstepping the background were considered to be labeled. In Fig. 3 the percentage of labeled cells

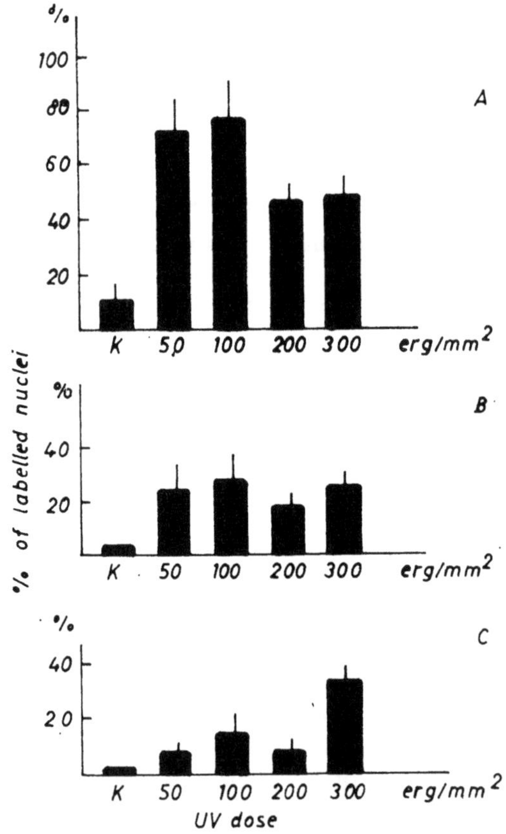

Fig. 3. Percentage of labeled lymphocytes after UV-irradiation, A — normal donor, B — XP II. C — classic XP.

immediately after exposure to UV-light is shown. At all doses, especially at dose of 10 J/m², the normal donor shows much higher percentage of labeled cells (nearby 80%), than both forms of XP (below 30%). Some decrease of unscheduled DNA synthesis at doses of 20 and 30 J/m² can be explained by the suppressing effect of higher doses of UV on repair process. These results are in agreement with other publications and show that XP II cells realize the decreased volume of UV-induced unscheduled DNA synthesis, as if classic XP cells.

We have also studied the unscheduled DNA synthesis induced by γ-rays. The lymphocyte cultures were irradiated with 50 and 100 krad doses of γ-rays. Conditions of experiment were the same as in UV-irradiation experiments. γ-irradiation causes much weaker unscheduled DNA synthesis than UV-irradiation does. If the unscheduled DNA synthesis really reflects repair replication, this phenomenon becomes understandable: gaps, induced by γ-rays are of 2—3 nucleotide extent, since UV-induced gaps after dimer excision and further degradation occur up to 100 nucleotides.

It is shown in Fig. 4 that 15—20% of cells of normal donor, as well as of classic XP

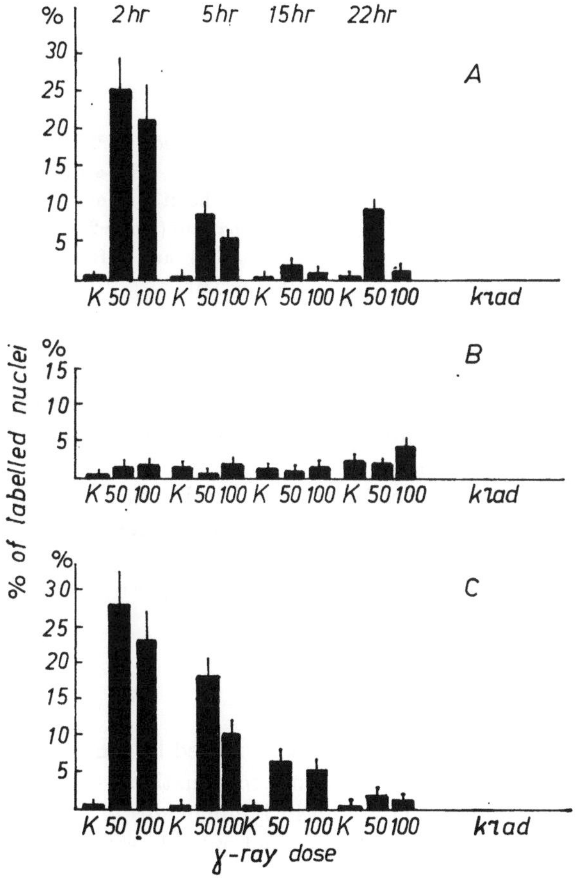

Fig. 4. Percentage of labeled lymphocytes at different time of incubation after γ-irradiation.

A — normal donor, B — XP II, C — classic XP.

(XP4LE) performe unscheduled DNA synthesis after γ-irradiation. Hence, the percentage of XP II cells, incorporating ^{3}H-thymidine, is only about 5%. Thus, the cells which are unable to rejoin γ-induced single-strand DNA breaks, perform also a considerably decreased, γ-induced unscheduled DNA synthesis. These data make more probable the defect in DNA-polymerase, which is necessary both for single-strand breaks rejoining and reparative synthesis performation in γ- and UV-irradiated cells.
The delayed DNA replication in XP2LE cells gives an additional evidence for DNA-polymerase defect in XP II. Fig. 5a shows ^{3}H-thymidine incorporation into lymphocyte nuclei as a function of incubation time after PHA stimulation of lymphocytes. The DNA synthesis in XP2LE cells is retarded as long as 5—6 hrs. It is of interest that UV-irradia-

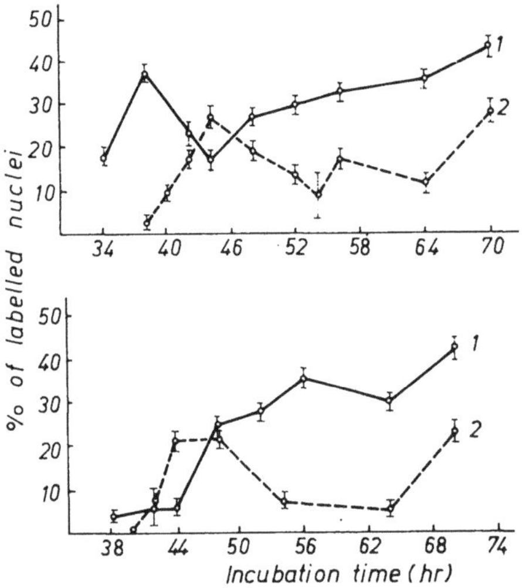

Fig. 5. Kinetics of ^{3}H-thymidine incorporation into PHA-stimulated lymphocytes of healthy donor (curve 1) and XP II patient (curve 2) without any irradiation (A) and after UV-irradiation 10 J/m^2 (B).

tion, which delays replication in normal lymphocytes, shows a negligible effect in XP II cells (Fig. 5b). Perhaps, UV-irradiation inhibits in normal cells the same factor, that is inhibited in XP II cells without irradiation.
Recently we have obtained data, that proliferation of XP2LE skin fibroblasts is delayed in comparison with that of normal fibroblasts and other XP lines we have. In addition, XP2LE fibroblasts undergo in culture a fewer number of generations than normal and other XP fibroblasts. So, in this respect XP II is similar to progeria, in which cells the γ-breaks DNA restitution is also defective.

Chromosomal effects in XP II cells

The data on the frequency of chromosome aberrations induced by ionizing radiation in XP cells are almost absent in the literature. The only information we know is a brief-mention in the work of Wolff (1968), who found in lymphocytes of 2 XP patients a little higher frequency of chromosome aberrations (not reliable statistically) than in normal cells.
In our experiments (Mikhelson, 1970; Mikhelson et al., 1974) lymphocytes of XP1LE, XP2LE, XP4LE, XPH2LE and normal donors were irradiated immediately after culture preparing, that is in G_0 phase of cell cycle at doses of 50, 100 and 150 R and then

incubated at +37° for 54—60 hrs. Metaphases were accumulated by colchicine, preparations were stained by Giemsa and metaphase plates were analysed microscopically.
We have found (Fig. 6) that there is no difference in the frequency of chromosome aberrations between cells of classic XP patients and normal ones. On the contrary, lymphocytes of the patient XP II were found to be reliably more sensitive (about 1.5 fold) than normal cells.
It is possible to draw an analogy between XP II and group of diseases with the syndrome of spontaneous chromosomal instability, in which cells the yield of X- and γ-induced chromosome aberrations is also increased, but to a greater degree than in XP II cells (Higurashi, Conen, 1973). So, in XP II and ataxia-telangiectasia cells there is some correlation between γ-damaged DNA repair defect and γ-induced chromosome

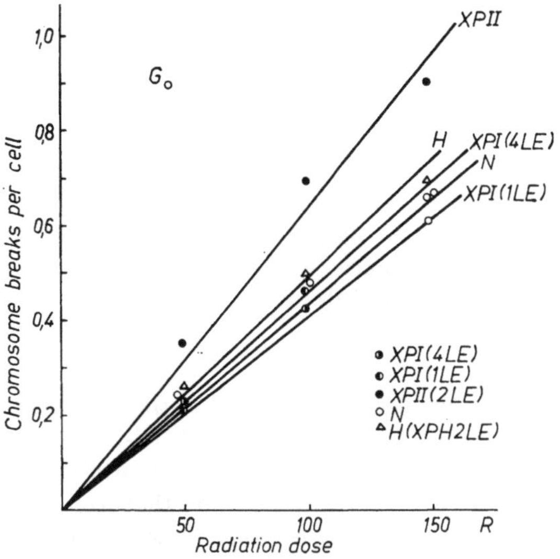

Fig. 6. Chromosome breaks frequency in γ-irradiated human lymphocytes of normal and XP donors.

aberrations yield. But in the most other cases such correlation is absent: in Bloom's-syndrome cells there is a very high level of γ-induced chromosome aberrations (Higurashi, Conen, 1973), but there is no defect in repair of γ-irradiated DNA (Kleijer, Bootsma, 1971); in Fanconi's-anemia cells there is the same picture (Fujivara, Tatsumi, 1975); in Hutchinson-Gilford progeria a very low level of γ-breaks repair is accompained by the normal frequency of γ-induced chromosome aberrations (Bender, Rary, 1974).
In our results the correlation between DNA repair and aberration yield in γ-irradiated cells is not complete too. If we believe that in the case of XP II the defect of rejoining of DNA breaks results in defect of chromosome rejoining, it is to be expected that the proportion of aberrations, requiring rejoining of broken chromosome ends in total yield of aberrations is to be smaller in the cells of XP II, than in normal cells. However we do not observe this. Figure 7 shows the percentage of such aberrations — dicentrics and rings — in the total number of aberrations. One can see that the percentage is approximately equal in the cells of patients with both forms of XP and in normal cells (the

total number of aberrations, and dicentrics and rings between them, in XP II cells is significantly higher).

These findings and similar results on other mutants with defective DNA repair allowed to form the hypothesis (Mikhelson, 1971) about the limited role of DNA repair in restitution of chromosomes, damaged by ionizing radiation. Recently this hypothesis has received a support in the works on the complicated structure of chromosomal DNA (Lett, 1976).

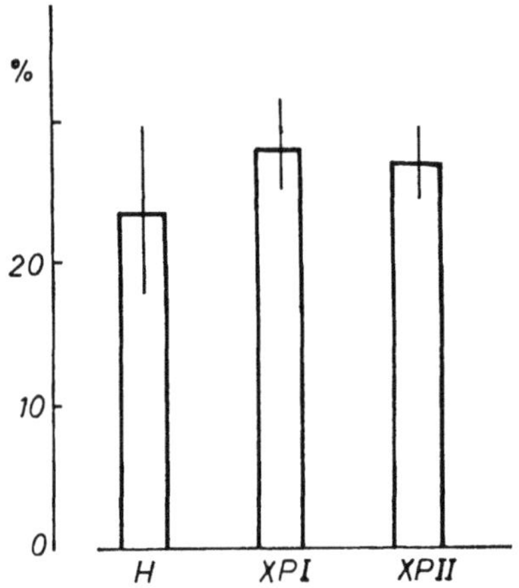

Fig. 7. The deal of aberrations, requiering rejoining of broken chromosome ends (rings and dicentrics) in the total yield of aberrations.

Frequency of UV-induced aberrations has been investigated in the lymphocytes of the same patients. The cells were irradiated by 5, 10 and 15 J/m² of UV-rays either immediately after culture prepairing — that is in G_0 phase of cell cycle — or after 12 hrs of incubation (G_1 phase), or after 48 hrs (G_2 phase). We can be sure that irradiation of lymphocytes immediately and after 12 hrs incubation corresponds respectively to phases

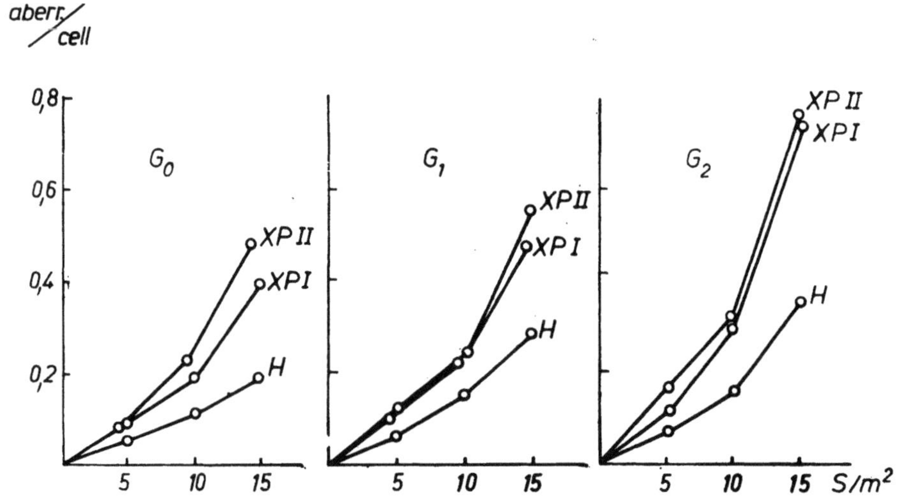

Fig. 8. Chromosome aberration frequency in UV-irradiated human lymphocytes of normal donor and XP patients in different studies of cell cycle.

G_0 and G_1, but as to the 48 hr, we can only speak of a predominance of cells in G_2 phase. Fig. 8 shows the dependence of aberration number per cell upon the dose of UV light in G_0, G_1 and G_2 phases of cycle. In all phases aberrations of chromatide type predominante. It is distinctly seen that at all phases the number of aberrations in cells of both XP forms is approximately twice as much as in normal cells. The difference between the two forms of XP is not reliable statistically.

In the Fig. 9 there is the comparison of the frequency of aberration in different phases of cell cycle at maximal dose (15 J/m²) in control normal cells (a), classic XP (b, left column) and XP II (b, right column). It is interesting to note that G_1 was found more

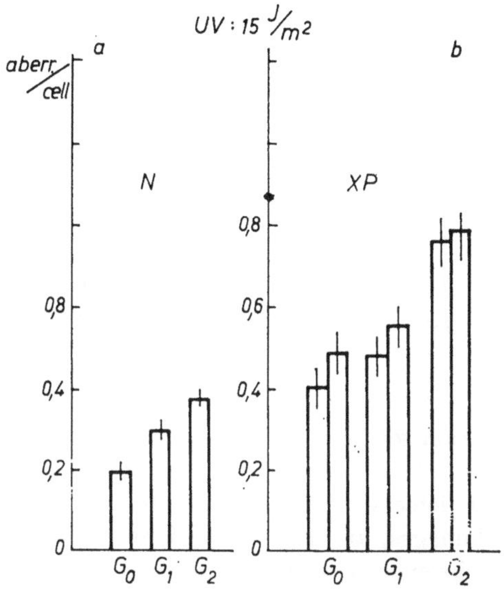

Fig. 9. Comparison of UV-induced aberration frequency in different phases of cell cycle in normal and XP lymphocytes.

sensitive to UV, than G_0, and the difference is retained in XP cells, defective in repair. So, this difference in radiosensitivity between cell cycle phases is not connected with excision repair of DNA.

On the whole, our results in UV-induced aberrations in XP are in agreement with the few data on classic XP, which are available in literature (PARRINGTON et al., 1971; MARSHALL, SCOTT, 1976). Chromosomes of XP II cells do not differ significantly from those of classic XP in UV-sensitivity.

To solve the problem of the role of DNA repair in normal vital functions of cell without any extreme treatment, it is of great interest to study spontaneous aberrations in the cells with repair defects. As I have already mentioned, the level of spontaneous aberrations in FANCONI's-anemia, ataxia-telangiectasia and BLOOM's-syndrome cells is sharply increased in comparison to normal cells. As to XP, there are very few and conflicting data. SASAKI (1973) found a little higher frequency of spontaneous aberrations in classic XP lymphocytes, but PARRINGTON et al. (1977) did not manage to show an increased level of spontaneous aberrations in XP fibroblasts.

We have investigated (MIKHELSON et al., 1976) the rate of spontaneous aberrations in the lymphocytes of our XP patients. In Fig. 10 the frequency of aberrations in intact lymphocytes of normal and XP donors is shown. The number of chromatide breaks per cell in XP of both forms is 2—3 fold higher, than in normal lymphocytes. For normal control cells it is 0.03 breaks per cell, for patients with classic XP — 0.08 (XP4LE) and 0.10 (XP1LE), and for XP II — 0.11 (XP2LE). Heterozygous XP II cells were also used as a control — 0.04 breaks per cell. Among spontaneous aberrations chromatide breaks (single fragments) predominate, and sometimes double fragments are met. We

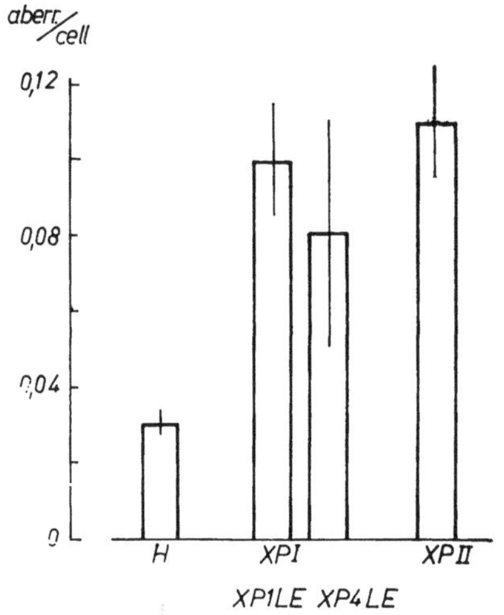

Fig. 10. Spontaneous chromosome aberration frequency in normal and XP lymphocytes.

do not see any difference in the aberration set between classic XP, XP II and normal lymphocytes.

The results obtained demonstrate that defects of enzyme systems, which are responsible for removal of DNA radiation damages, are accompanied by an increase of the frequency of spontaneous damages of chromosomes. This confirms the idea of community of enzyme systems involved in repair of hereditary structures in the course of normal vital functions and under extreme treatments (Paribok, 1965; Zhestyanikov, 1974).

Role of defective DNA repair in carcinogenesis and aging

All the known diseases with defective DNA repair, except progeria, are characterized by high frequency of chromosome damage and increased risk of malignization. On the other hand, progeria and less the other diseases — Fanconi's-anemia, Bloom's-syndrome, ataxia-telangiectasia — are characterized by the premature aging and shortened lifespan of both patients and cells in vitro. It makes one search for the cause of aging and malignization in defective DNA repair.

Theories of aging and carcinogenesis based on the accumulation of genetic damage are known long ago (Burnet, 1957; Szilard, 1959; Yielding, 1974). According to these theories, on the one hand, the accumulation of damage in DNA gradually decrease the functional abilities with age; on the other, damage in critical regions of the genome can lead to somatic mutations resulting in malignization. Hayflick's-data (Hayflick, Moorhead, 1961; Hayflick, 1965; 1967; 1975) about limited potential of somatic cell division give experimental evidence for these theories.

Close correlation observed between the mutagenic and carcinogenic activity of many agents makes it possible to suggest that unrepaired or defectively repaired DNA damage can result in mutagenesis, and that mutation in certain regions of the genome is the cause of carcinogenesis. In this case one can expect an increased frequency of both spontaneous and induced somatic mutations in diseases with defective DNA repair.

The frequency of somatic mutations induced by UV-radiation and some chemical carcinogens has been studied only in XP. It has been shown (Maher, 1973; 1975; 1976; 1977) that UV-light and chemical carcinogens sharply increase azaguanidine resistance mutation rate in cultured fibroblasts of classical and "variant" forms of XP, compared with effect of the same agents in normal fibroblasts. This is of course a serious confirmation of the somatic mutation theory of cancer.

The other illustration of high mutation level in XP is Burnet's-hypothesis which considers the skin freckles as a result of mutations. According to this theory (Burnet, 1970) all the freckles in normal and XP patient skin represent clones of melanocytes, originating from a single melanocyte that had undergone a UV-induced mutation. So, the excessive number of freckles in the skin of XP patients might be the result of the increased mutation rate, arising from the faulty repair of DNA (Lutzner, Scott, 1971). In this way hypo- and depigmented areas in the skin of XP patients could be explained as a consequence of the appearance of albino-type melanocytes on account of mutation (Fitzpatrick, Quevado, 1972; Robbins et al., 1974).

Experimental data on the frequency of somatic mutations in other diseases with DNA repair defect are not available.

Data on classic XP give little support for aging theories based on repair processes, as neither XP cells in vitro (except cells of XP II patient) nor XP patients show premature aging. Incidently, death of XP patients at early age can to a certain extent mask slight premature aging. Besides, the progressive loss of neurons in the neurological form of XP is age related.

Studies of progeria give much more material in this respect. The attempts to find a correlation between cell age and the efficiency of repair processes, as well as between life span and the relative amount of repair have not given unquestionable results up to now (Cleaver, Bootsma, 1975; Setlow, 1974). Progeria cells give the first example of an obvious correlation between defective DNA repair, rapid aging of cells in vitro, and premature aging in vivo. Preliminary results on other diseases (XP II, ataxia-telangiectasia) allow such correlation to be expected. It can be mentioned here the data on lower molecular weight of unirradiated DNA observed in XP II (Mikhelson et al., 1974) and progeria (Little et al., 1974) in comparison to that of normal cells.

In conclusion it should be said that XP and other repair defective human and not only human mutants is still a fruitful field of investigation as a model system for repair mechanisms of DNA and chromosomes, carcinogenesis and related problems. The search for other repair deficient mutants is our important purpose.

References

[1] Arlett, C. F.: Mutat. Res., **46**, 106 (1977)
[2] Bender, M. A., Rary, J. M.: Radiat. Res. **59**, 181 (1974)
[3] Bloom, D.: Arch. Derm. Syph. **69**, 526 (1954)
[4] Brown, W. T., Epstein, J., Little, J. B.: Exper. Cell. Res. **97**, 291 (1976)

[5] Burk, P., Yuspa, S., Lutzner, M., Robbins, J.: Lancet **1**, 7799, 601 (1971)
[6] Burnet, M.: Brit. Med. J. **6**, 779 (1957)
[7] Burnet, M. 1970. In: Immunologic Surveillance, NY, Pergamon Press 50
[8] Cleaver, J. E.: Nature **218**, 652 (1968)
[9] Cleaver, J. E.: Proc. Nat. Acad. Sci. USA **63**, 428 (1969)
[10] Cleaver, J. E.: Intern. J. Rad. Biol. **18**, 557 (1970)
[11] Cleaver, J. E.: J. Invest. Dermatol. **58**, 124 (1972)
[12] Cleaver, J. E., Bootsma, D.: Ann. Rev. Genetics **9**, 19 (1975)
[13] Cleaver, J. E., Bootsma, D., Friedberg, E. C.: Genetics **79**, suppl. II, 215 (1975)
[14] Emerit, J., Housset, E., Groushy, J. de, Camus, J. P.: Rev. Europ. Etud. Clin. Biol. **16**, 684 (1971)
[15] Emerit, J., Levi, A., Housset, E.: Humangenetik **25**, 221 (1974)
[16] Epstein, J. H., Williams, J. R., Little, J. B.: Proc. Nat. Acad. Sci. USA **70**, 977 (1973)
[17] Epstein, J. H., Williams, J. R., Little, J. B.: Biochem. Biophys. Res. Comm. **59**, 850 (1974)
[18] Fanconi, G.: Jb. Kinderheilk. Phys. Erzieh. **117**, 257 (1927)
[19] Fitzpatrick, T., Quevado, W. 1972. In: Initial Metabol. Basis Inher. Dis. NY, 326
[20] Fujivara, Y., Tatsumi, M.: Biochem. Biophys. Res. Comm. **66**, 592 (1975)
[21] Gilford, H.: Practitioner **53**, 188 (1904)
[22] Goht, K., Cleaver, J. E.: Radiat. Res. **62**, 581 (1975)
[23] Goldstein, S.: Lancet **1**, 7591, 424 (1969)
[24] Goldstein, S.: Proc. Soc. Exp. Biol. Med. **137**, 730 (1971)
[25] Hayflick, L.: Exper. Cell. Res. **37**, 614 (1965)
[26] Hayflick, L.: Nat. Cancer Inst. Monogr. **26**, 355 (1967)
[27] Hayflick, L.: Federat. Proc. **37**, 9 (1975)
[28] Hayflick, L., Moorhead, P. S.: Exp. Cell Res. **25**, 585 (1961)
[29] Haykazyan, E. V., Mikhelson, V. M., Zhestianikov, V. D.: Tsitologia **15**, 881 (1973)
[30] Heiner, L.: Orvosi Hetilap **69**, 540 (1925)
[31] Higurashi, M., Conen, P. E.: Cancer **32**, 380 (1973)
[32] Hutchinson, J. 1886 Cite for: Gilford H., 1904.
[33] Jung, E. G.: Nature **228**, 361 (1970)
[34] Jung, E. G.: Dermatologica (Basel) **142**, 269 (1971)
[35] Jung, E. G.: Hautarzt. **24**, 175 (1973)
[36] Kleijer, W. J., Bootsma, D.: In: Proc. 1st Europ. Biophys. Congr., Baden **2**, 129 (1971)
[37] Kleijer, W. J., Lohman, P. H. M., Mulder, M. P., Bootsma, D.: Mutat. Res. **9**, 517 (1970)
[38] Lambert, B., Ringborg, U., Swanbeck, G. Mutat. Res., **46**, 133 (1977)
[39] Lehmann, A. R., Kirk-Bell, S., Arlett, C. F., Paterson, M. C., Lohman, P. H. M., Weerd-Kastelein, E. A. de, Bootsma, D.: Proc. Nat. Acad. Sci. USA **72**, 219 (1975)
[40] Lett, J. T. 1976. In: Aging, Carcinogenesis a. Rad. Biology, 11
[41] Little, J. B., Epstein, J., Williams, J. R. 1974. In: Molec. Mech. Repair DNA, Irvine-California, 9
[42] Louis-Bar, D.: Confin. Neurol. (Basel) **4**, 32 (1941)
[43] Lutzner, M. A., Scott, C. I.: Birth Defects. **7**, 296 (1971)
[44] Maher, V. M., Wessel, G., McCormick, J. J.: J. Cell Biol. **59**, 213a (1973)
[45] Maher, V. M., Mishke, B. S., McCormick, J. J.: Proc. Nat. Acad. Sci. USA **72**, 72 (1975)
[46] Maher, V. M., Quelette, L. M., Gurren, R. D., McCormick, J. J.: Nature **261**, 593 (1976)
[47] Maher, V. M., McCormick, J. J. Mutat. Res., **46**, 139 (1977)
[48] Marshall, R. R., Scott, D.: Mutat. Res. **36**, 397 (1976)
[49] Martenstein, H., Bobowitcz, A.: Arch. Dermat. Syph. **150**, 165 (1926)
[50] Mikhelson, V. M. 1970. In: Mater. Scient. Conf. Inst. Cytol., Leningrad, 57
[51] Mikhelson, V. M.: Tsitologia **13**, 932 (1971)
[52] Mikhelson, V. M., Haykazyan, E. V.: Doklady Akad. Nauk SSSR **206**, 1462 (1972)

[53] MIKHELSON, V. M., HAYKAZYAN, E. V., GENTER, E. I., PLESKACH, N. M.: Tsitologia **16**, 203 (1974)
[54] MIKHELSON, V. M., SLONIMSKAYA, E. I., PROKOFIEVA, V. V., ZHESTYANIKOV, V. D.: Doklady Akad. Nauk SSSR **230**, 965 (1976)
[55] MÜLLER, W., YAMAZAKI, Z., ZAHN, R., BREHM, G., KORTING, G.: Biochem. Biophys. Res. Comm. **44**, 433 (1971)
[56] PARIBOK, V. P.: Radiobiologia (Inf. bull.) **7**, 38 (1965)
[57] PARRINGTON, J. M., DELHANTY, D. A., BADEN, H. P.: Ann. Human Genet. **35**, 149 (1971)
[58] PARRINGTON, J. M., CASEY, G., WEST, L., VASCONCELOS MAIA, V. DE. Mutat. Res., **46**, 146 (1977)
[59] PASSARGE, E.: Humangenetik **16**, 151 (1972)
[60] PATERSON, M. C. Mutat. Res., **46**, 148 (1977)
[61] PATERSON, M. C., SMITH, B. R., KNIGHT, P. A., ANDERSON, A. K. 1977. In: Proc. VII Intern. Congr. on Photobiol., Rome, 1
[62] POON, P. K., O'BRIEN, R. L., PARKER, J. W.: Nature **250**, 223 (1974)
[63] REGAN, J. D., SETLOW, R. B.: Cancer Res. **34**, 3318 (1974)
[64] ROBBINS, J. H., KRAEMER, K. H., LUTZNER, M. A., FESTOFF, B. W., GOON, H. G.: Ann. Intern. Med. **80**, 221 (1974)
[65] SASAKI, M. S.: Mutat. Res. **20**, 291 (1973)
[66] SCHROEDER, T. M., TILGEN, D., KRUGER, J., VOGEL, F.: Humangenetik **32**, 257 (1976)
[67] SETLOW, R. B. 1974. In: Mol. Mechanisms of Repair of DNA, NY, 711
[68] SHANIN, A. P. 1952. Malignant tumors, Leningrad. "Medicina"
[69] SHANIN, A. P. 1969. Skin tumors and its origin. Leningrad. "Medicina"
[70] SZILARD, L.: Proc. Nat. Acad. Sci. USA, **45**, 30 (1959)
[71] TANAKA, K., SEKIGUCHI, M., OKADA, Y.: Proc. Nat. Acad. Sci. USA **72**, 4071 (1975)
[72] WEERD-KASTELEIN, E. A. DE, KEIJZER, W., BOOTSMA, D. 1972. Nature New Biolog **238**, 80 (1972)
[73] WEERD-KASTELEIN, E. A. DE, KEIJZER, W., SABOUR, M., PARRINGTON, J. M., BOOTSMA, D. Mutat. Res., **46**, 163 (1977)
[74] WADE, M., CHU, E., SCHMICKEL, R. Mutat. Res., **46**, 162 (1977)
[75] WOLFF, S., SCOTT, D.: Exp. Cell Res. **55**, 9 (1968)
[76] YIELDING, K. L.: Perspect. Biol. Med. **17**, 201 (1974)
[77] ZHESTYANIKOV, V. D.: Radiobiologia (Inform. bull.) **16**, 5 (1974)

CLINICAL ASPECTS OF DNA REPAIR

The Importance of Frame-Shift Mutations in Carcinogenesis

W. Presber and D. H. Krüger

Chair of Virology, 104 Berlin, Schumannstr. 20/21, GDR

Up to this day the molecular mechanisms of carcinogenesis are unresolved. This is reflected by overwhelming numbers of theories and hypotheses.

Despite elaborate research in this field it isn't even clear whether the genetic information for cancer is already present in every cell or not (Temin, 1972; Temin, 1974a; Todaro and Huebner, 1972; Lieber et al., 1975; Gallo et al., 1974; Spiegelman, 1974).

We cannot attempt to solve this controversy but would like to propose a molecular mechanism which encompasses several hypotheses and which reconciles certain contradictions.

Our point of departure is the fact that in a cancer cell or in a transformed cell new specific genome sections are expressed, i.e., that cancer is a problem of the cell's molecular regulation. This "sudden" expression can have several causes, for example:

— the cancer genes or parts of them were newly introduced into the cell by a virus.
— the cancer genes were there all the time and had to be activated by chemical or physical cancerogens or by viruses (Temin, 1974a).

In this connection it is irrelevant and impossible to assess whether this cancer information is of cellular origin or whether it was introduced by a virus but not immediately expressed. In any case the realization of the cancer information can be explained by a common molecular event: a frame-shift mutation.

In the following we will discuss this mechanism.

Chemical mutagenesis

We know for a long time that a multitude of chemicals can cause cancer (Brookes, 1975). While not all mutagens are carcinogens, the reverse seems to be true: all carcinogens are mutagens (McCann et al., 1975).

Are carcinogens a special class of mutagens? Recently a number of papers appeared about carcinogens which induce frameshift mutations (McCann et al., 1975; Ames et al., 1973; Isono and Yourno, 1974; Roth, 1974). Although one should not overemphasize these first results — the number of substances tested was limited, the test systems (bacterial mutants) hardly resemble higher organisms, and the mechanisms of action were usually not clear (Roth, 1974) — we shall discuss their implications.

Frame-shift mutations can have two essentially different results:

1. Genetic information mutates out-of-frame and can no longer be expressed.
2. Out-of-frame information restores its expressibility by a new frame-shift mutation.

Since eukaryote cells contain a substantial amount of redundant DNA (Ohno, 1971) which is not expressed and therefore neither subject to control nor selection it is conceivable that large DNA sections are mutated out-of-frame without any consequences for the organism. An activation of these genes at some later point by frame-shift mutation may heavily interfere with normal cellular regulation and lead to cancer. Such usually not expressed sections which are only "revived" by frame-shift, correspond to Temin's "new DNA sequences" and his models number 3 and 4, which postulate that integration of viruses leads to expression of previously inaccessible cellular information (Temin, 1974a).

Naturally the expression of cancer information depends on functional promotors and other regulatory sequences. Intercistronic buffer sequences (Frontali and Morpurgo,

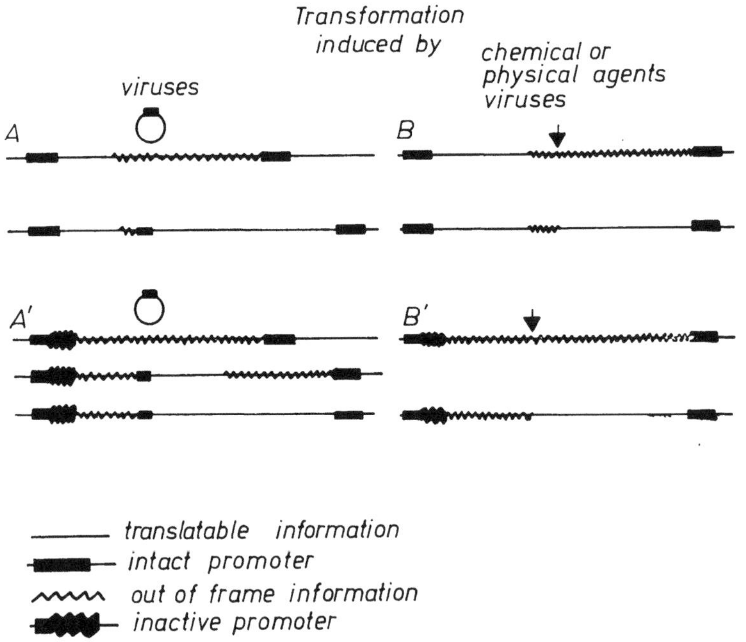

1972) ensure that only a limited area of the chromosome becomes untranslatable or translatable again following a frame-shift mutation, i.e. the changes in gene expression are not excessive (Fig., part A and B).

This hypothesis of gene activation by frame-shift explains how cells of one clone can be differently transformed by one and the same cancerogen (Prehn, 1968; Mondat et al., 1970) – the differences showing up as "tumour antigen" and serologically. The activation simply takes place at different parts of the genome, and, depending on which gene was activated, different antigens appear (Embleton and Heidelberger, 1972). Transformation without new antigens would mean that the frameshift activation did not occur in a pertinent gene.

This explanation of chemical carcinogenesis by frame-shift mutations is also valid for virus-induced malignant transformation.

Viral carcinogenesis

In classical transformation, the virus enters a cell and with a certain probability its genome is integrated into the cell genome and the cell is transformed (TEMIN, 1974b; ECKHART, 1974). Already in 1971 ZINDER suggested that a mutation which may occur during the integration of tumour virus DNA is the true cause of carcinogenesis. This is most probably a frame-shift mutation which alters the reading frame of those host sequences which are located next to the virus genome or its promoter (see below and Fig. part A and A').

Meanwhile it was shown that the integration of virus DNA is necessary for cellular transformation (HILL et al., 1974). In analogy to chemical carcinogenesis, a frame-shift mutation which occurs during integration with high probability, renders out-of-frame information of the host readable (Fig. part A and A'). This would explain how viral carcinogenesis can take place without involvement of virus information (also by small tumour virus fragments) (see for review GALLO and LEVINE, 1974) and also, why not every integration of a tumour virus leads to malignant growth (BOETTINGER, 1974) — because the reading frame was not altered. Evidence that UV-inactivated viruses can sometimes transform puts forth the question, whether in some cases integration and the resulting mutation alone are enough to induce carcinogenesis.

Besides these features that viral carcinogenesis has in common with chemical carcinogenesis, there are a number of peculiarities:

1. Tumour viruses introduce their own functional promoter and regulation sites, which increase the probability of expression of genome sequences already present in the cell. It has been shown that sometimes at the beginning of virus-specific protein synthesis only a part of the virus genome is transcribed, but the mRNA is much longer and contains cellular sequences as well (HIRT, 1973; WALL and DARNELL, 1971; TSUEI et al., 1972). In this connection HOBOM (HOBOM, 1973) discusses the possible significance of normally silent host genes in carcinogenesis, and suggests that a small virus may only supply a strong promoter inducing the expression of silent genes which disturb normal cellular regulation.
2. Tumour viruses are often very specific regarding their attachment and integration sites, which would enable specific activation of certain sequences.
3. Viruses in general and also tumour viruses have their own "regulation systems" or can modify those of the host. Functions of this kind were termed pleiotropic effectors by WEIL et al. (WEIL et al., 1974). Thus virus-specific functions (like methylases) can influence the expression of host genes, if for instance the methylation (modification) pattern of certain sequences is altered so that they evade normal regulation (theory of aberrant methylation (see GANTT, 1974); for recent results on possible methylation dependence of gene expression see KRÜGER et al. (KRÜGER et al., 1975)). It is conceivable that this alone could lead to malignant growth.

Such pleiotropic virus functions may be affected in the well-known SV40 and adenovirus ts mutants, since the temperature-sensitive alteration varies with the cell type (see for review ECKHART, 1974). Since the transformation is not completely reversible following temperature-shift there may be other changes involved, possibly frame-shift mutations.

If a virus was integrated without frame-shift and has no function that interferes with the host's gene expression, infection proceeds without transformation. However, such "silent" proviruses can be induced by chemicals like BUdR (Jacob and Wollmann, 1953) or by radiation (Gerber, 1972) and then reproduce "lytically", the progeny viruses infecting other cells and now integrating out of frame. In this way, frame-shift mutations are produced indirectly by agents that are not themselves frame-shift mutagens.

Physical carcinogenesis

Following our model, radiation acts as a carcinogen by causing primary DNA lesions which induce repair processes. During repair, frame-shift mutations could occur. Furthermore these repair processes lead to a high frequency of virus integration (Seemayer and Defendi, 1973) and therefore frame-shifts.
A release of integrated viruses could also reverse the frame-shift mutation and thus the transformed state of the cell. This means that effective cancerostatic agents with the ability to reverse the transformation process are probably frame-shift mutagens and are cancerostatic and cancerogenous at the same time. This was shown to be the case for a number of cancerostatics (Beal et al., 1975).

Concluding remarks

Frame-shift mutations, as well as methylation (and other modifications, like the incorporation of BUdR or IUdR into DNA), cause changes in gene expression (also changes of an already transformed state (Davidson and Horn, 1974)). Probably such processes interact. The effect of frame-shift mutations alone could be distinguished experimentally from the other processes through the fact that repair processes are always involved, and also by inducing specific reversions of frame-shift mutations.
The purpose of this article was to suggest new experimental approaches for the elucidation of carcinogenesis.

References

[1] Ames, B. N., Dursten, W. E., Yamasaki, E., Lee, F. D.: Proc. Natl. Acad. Sci. USA **70**, 2281–2285 (1973)
[2] Beal, D. D., Skibba, J. L., Croft, W. A., Cohen, S. M., Bryan, G. T.: J. Natl. Canc. Inst. **54**, 951–957 (1975)
[3] Boettinger, D.: Cell **3**, 71–76 (1974)
[4] Brookes, P.: Life Sciences **16**, 331–344 (1975)
[5] Davidson, R. L., Horn, D.: Proc. Natl. Acad. Sci. USA **71**, 3338–3342 (1974)
[6] Eckhardt, W.: Annu. Rev. Genetics **8**, 301–317 (1974)
[7] Embleton, M. J., Heidelberger, C.: Internat. J. Canc. **9**, 8–18 (1972)
[8] Frontali, L., Morpurgo, G. J.: J. theor. Biol. **36**, 147–151 (1972)
[9] Gallo, R. C., Levine, A.: Cell **2**, 295–304 (1974)
[10] Gallo, R. C., Gallagher, R. E., Ting, R. C., Smith, R. G., Gillispie, D. H., Wu, A. M.: Cancer Chemotherapy Reports part I, **58**, 579–593 (1974)
[11] Gannt, R. R.: J. Natl. Canc. Inst. **53**, 1505–1508 (1974)

[12] Gerber, P.: Proc. Natl. Acad. Sci. USA **69**, 83—85 (1972)
[13] Hill, M., Hillova, J., Dantchev, D., Mariage, R., Goubin, G.: Cold Spring Harb. Symp. Quant. Biol. **XXXIX**, 1015—1025 (1974)
[14] Hirt, B.: Path. Microbiol. **39**, 24—31 (1973)
[15] Hobom, G.: Biol. in unserer Zeit **3**, 87—93 (1973)
[16] Isono, K., Yourno, J.: Proc. Natl. Acad. Sci. USA **71**, 1612—1617 (1974)
[17] Jacob, F., Wollmann, E. L.: Cold Spring Harb. Symp. Quant. Biol. **18**, 101—120 (1953)
[18] Krüger, D. H., Presber, W., Hansen, S., and Rosenthal, H. A.: J. Virology **16**, 453—455 (1975)
[19] Lieber, M. M., Beneviste, R. E., Livingston, D. M., Todaro, G. J.: Science **182**, 56—58 (1975)
[20] McCann, J., Spingarn, N. E., Kobori, J., Ames, B. N.: Proc. Natl. Acad. Sci. USA **72**, 979—983 (1975)
[21] Mondat, S., Iype, P. T., Griesbach, L. M., Heidelberger, C.: Cancer Res. **30**, 1593—1597 (1970)
[22] Ohno, S.: Nature **234**, 134—137 (1971)
[23] Prehn, R. T.: Cancer Res. **28**, 1326—1330 (1968)
[24] Roth, J. R.: Annu. Rev. Genetics 8, 319—346 (1974)
[25] Seemayer, N. M., Defendi, V.: Virology **12**, 1265—1271 (1973)
[26] Spiegelman, S.: Cancer Chemotherapy Reports part I, **58**, 595—613 (1974)
[27] Temin, H. M.: Proc. Natl. Acad. Sci. USA **69**, 1016—1020 (1972)
[28] Temin, H. M.: Cancer **34**, 1347—1352 (1974a)
[28] Temin, H. M.: Annu. Rev. Genetics 8, 155—177 (1974b)
[30] Todaro, G. J., Huebner, R. J.: Proc. Natl. Acad. Sci. USA **69**, 1009—1015 (1972)
[31] Tsuei, D., Fujinaga, K., Green, M.: Proc. Natl. Acad. Sci. USA **69**, 427—430 (1972)
[32] Wall, R., Darnell, J. E.: Nature New Biol. **232**, 13—26 (1971)
[33] Weil, R., Salomon, C., May, E., May, P.: Cold Spring Harb. Symp. Quant. Biol. **XXXIX**, 381—395 (1974)
[34] Zinder, N. B., 1971, Perspectives in Virology VIII (Acad. Press, New York—London) pp 15 to 22

Clinical Aspects of DNA Repair

R. J. Wilkins

University of Otago Medical School, Dunedin, New Zealand.

1. Introduction

Research into human DNA repair mechanisms has now advanced to the stage where significant medical applications can be expected within the next decade. Perhaps the most exciting of these potential applications is that of testing patients for DNA repair capacity and thus obtaining information which will complement the conventional procedures for the diagnosis and prognosis of cancerous conditions. Indeed, limited use of such tests has already been made. What is needed now is to view the medical relevance of DNA repair mechanisms with a much widened perspective.

Several criteria have to be met before DNA repair capacity can be regarded as a clinically useful parameter. We must first of all appreciate the levels of cellular DNA damage that repair mechanisms have to cope with. That is, we must have good estimates of the DNA damage induced by various environmental agents — both natural and artificial. Second, we must estimate the capacity of repair mechanisms to deal with this damage. Third, in those cases where DNA repair is deficient, we need to seek correlations with various clinical features in the patient. Fourth, we need to ascertain whether or not there is a range of repair capacities in "normal" humans and if any small deficiencies in repair predisposes the individual to some of the symptoms seen in patients with gross deficiencies in repair. Lastly, a simple and reliable test is required which will give parameters of DNA repair capacity which are easy to interpret clinically. As yet, such tests are not available.

These criteria will be discussed in the following sections. The aim will be to establish a clinical perspective rather than to review an extensive literature which makes largely incidental reference to medical aspects of DNA repair.

2. The Environment and DNA Damage

A realistic assessment of the role of DNA repair mechanisms is only possible if one is familiar with the levels of DNA damage which arise from environmental sources. Unfortunately, virtually all laboratory experiments are quite unrealistic in this respect. One only has to compare the massive doses of ionising radiations or chemical carcinogens which are used experimentally with the levels found in nature to realise the extent of these differences. In the case of x-rays, experimental doses are often several krad whereas the natural background radiation dose to humans is only about 100 mrad per year; similarly, for the carcinogen N-dimethylnitrosamine the experimental doses may be millimolar (San and Stich, 1975) yet natural sources (Montesano and Bartsch, 1976) are unlikely to give rise to concentrations of greater than micromolar in the body. In general, experimental conditions measure the ability of DNA repair systems to cope with extreme challenges rather than measuring their performance under natural conditions. This point is often overlooked.

The following examples illustrate the range of DNA damage which can be induced in the human body by environmental agents.

The most ubiquitous damage arises from the physiological conditions inside the living cell. LINDAHL and NYBERG (1972) estimate that at 37 °C depurination sites form in the DNA of a human cell at the rate of about 10 per minute. The exact biological significance of these sites is debatable, with DRAKE and BALTZ (1976) concluding that depurination is not a mechanism for mutagenesis, while KUHNLEIN, PENHOET and LINN (1976) imply that defective repair of apurinic sites may give rise to the neurological disorders associated with Xeroderma pigmentosum. DRAKE and BALTZ suggest that "heat" mutagenesis may be the result of the transmigration of N-glycosidic bonds in DNA and that this could induce 0.07 potential mutations per minute per human cell at 37 °C. Whatever the exact mechanism of DNA induction by physiological conditions, it is clear that the magnitude of the damage is such to demand efficient repair.

In contrast to intracellular conditions, the contribution made to DNA damage by natural background radiation seems, at first glance, to be extremely small. Thus, a background dose rate of 100 mrad per year may only damage an average of one DNA base per million cells per minute (assuming a G-value for damage to bases of about 2; DERTINGER and JUNG, 1970). This analysis is, however, grossly oversimplified as it ignores the fact that the dose from ionising radiations is not distributed uniformly throughout tissue. On a microdosimetric scale it can be shown (KELLERER, 1976) that a small fraction of cells in the body will have very large doses deposited in their sensitive volumes no matter how low the average radiation dose. These microdoses may vary from a few rad to hundreds of rad, depending on the quality of the radiation, and they will produce some 10 to 1000 lesions in the DNA of a "hit" cell nucleus. Thus, no matter how low the average dose to the body, and no matter how minimal the overall damage, there will always be an occasional cell in which quite substantial quantities of DNA damage will have to be repaired. Moreover, as mammalian cells can be transformed in vitro by neutron doses of at least as low as 100 mrad (BOREK, 1976) it is reasonable to assume that damage to isolated cells could be biologically important.

Solar UV radiation is perhaps the most potent of all environmental agents which damage DNA. Exposure to summer sunlight in temperate latitudes has been estimated to produce DNA damage in the upper dermis of untanned Caucasian skin at the same rate as would $2\ J \cdot m^{-2} \cdot h^{-1}$ of 254 nm light (WILKINS, 1974); the corresponding number of cyclobutane pyrimidine dimers induced in the DNA of a human cell is about 1.300 per minute! Furthermore, when one recalls that the D_{37} dose for human cells is only about $4\ J \cdot m^{-2}$ (CLEAVER and BOOTSMA, 1975), it is clear that this damage is several orders of magnitude greater than that induced by most other environmental agents. Of course, UV light only damages the skin. Nevertheless, the probability of one unrepaired dimer producing a neoplastic transformation may be of the order of 10^{-10} (SETLOW and HART, 1975; CHAN and LITTLE, 1976) so it follows that, in human skin exposed to moderate sunlight, the potential transformation rate could be of the order of 10^{-5} per hour. Such a transformation rate could not be tolerated (CAIRNS, 1975) and repair mechanisms would have to intervene.

From these examples it is clear that there are large differences in the magnitudes of environmentally induced DNA damage. Solar UV is among the most damaging of all environmental sources and thus it is no surprise that Caucasians suffer a high incidence of skin cancers and that this incidence varies with UV exposure (Emmett, 1973). Moreover, because this damage places such demands on DNA repair systems it is hardly surprising that a Xeroderma pigmentosum patient who is grossly defective in the repair of such damage is going to develop early and extensive solar induced skin cancers. In contrast, the levels of DNA damage induced by other environmental agents are unlikely to be high enough for the consequences of defective repair to be so obvious. For example, in the disease ataxia telangiectasia which has been described as an "ionizing radiation counterpart of Xeroderma pigmentosum" (Paterson et al., 1976) the radiosensitivity of patients only becomes obvious when they are exposed to radiotherapy level doses; background radiation doses are simply too low to give symptoms analogous to those seen in Xeroderma pigmentosum.

3. Normal and Defective DNA Repair Mechanisms

Before describing diseases which are characterised by defective DNA repair, it is worth outlining in quantitative terms just what is meant by "normal" and "defective" repair capacity. Unless otherwise stated, the results quoted below pertain to cultured human cells.

(*i*) *Excision Repair*

Excision repair is the most extensively studied of all repair processes and it is now believed to operate on a wide range of DNA damage. For example, on pyrimidine dimers induced by UV-light, on endonuclease-sensitive-sites induced by ionising radiation and on purine adducts (Q.Pu) induced by 4-nitroquinoline-1-oxide (4NQO). The rates at which these lesions can be removed from cells suffering substantial damage are all strikingly similar — somewhere between one and two thousand lesions per minute per cell. In the case of UV light (Paterson, Lohman and Sluyter, 1973) this rate is comparable to that at which sunlight induces damage in human skin, whereas in the cases of both ionising radiation (Paterson et al., 1976) and 4NQO (Ikenaga et al., 1975), the excision rates are greatly in excess of the rates of induction of environmental damage. These investigators find defective excision rates of UV damage in Xeroderma pigmentosum cells (one-third to one-tenth normal), of γ-ray damage in some ataxia telangiectasia cells (about one-third normal) and of Q.Pu damage in Xeroderma pigmentosum cells (about one-fifth normal). The values quoted above are for the *initial* rates of excision; there appears to be a much larger fraction of repair resistant damage at later times in repair deficient than in repair proficient cells and this damage can persist for many days (e.g. Wilkins, 1973).

Excision repair is a complex enzymatic process, but it is tempting to postulate that the major differences in both the repair of different types of DNA lesions and in the various repair deficiencies, lie in the initial incision step. That is to say, specific endonucleases recognise specific classes of lesions and the impairment of the function of one of these endonucleases leads to an observable defect in excision repair. As a corollary, one would

expect a common pathway for the remaining steps of excision repair which would function in both normal and excision deficient cells. Indeed, such has been shown to be the case in Xeroderma pigmentosum cells (Cook et al., 1975).
The implications are twofold if the major defects in excision repair occur at the incision step. First, detection of such defects is simplified because we need only test the ability of cells to make single-strand breaks in damaged DNA. Second, damage which is not excised should remain in a form which is amenable to postreplication repair processes (Hastings, Quah and von Borstel, 1976).

(*ii*) *Postreplication Repair*

Postreplication repair is the subject of increasing investigation (Lehmann, 1974) partly because it is believed to be a more error prone process than excision repair and thus may be important in mutagenesis and carcinogenesis. Unlike excision repair, postreplication repair bypasses rather than removes DNA lesions. The efficiency of this mechanism is difficult to estimate but it does appear to enable in excess of 10.000 unexcised dimers to be tolerated in an UV-irradiated cell (Lehmann, 1974). Defective postreplication repair has been observed in the variant class of Xeroderma pigmentosum patients whom appear proficient in the excision of dimers but nevertheless develop the main symptoms of the disease. Cells cultured from these patients are now known to be slow in converting the daughter DNA synthesized after UV-irradiation into a high molecular weight form; this conversion process is also strongly inhibited by caffeine (Lehmann et al., 1975). Some classical Xeroderma pigmentosum cells show limited evidence of this defect, but it has not been observed in cells of patients suffering from ataxia telangiectasia, Fanconi's-anemia, progeria, "sunlight sensitivity" or multiple carcinomas (Lehmann, Kirk-Bell and Arlett, 1976).
A bewildering array of models and mechanisms have been postulated to account for postreplication repair processes. While not attempting to add to this confusion, some comment is necessary. The most important point to be made is that moderate sunlight exposures induce many tens of thousands of dimers in the cells of human skin and *regardless* of the presence or absence of an excision repair system, most of these dimers will remain in the DNA for several hours after exposure during which time they must be susceptible to the postreplication repair processes. What then, protects normal cells (and humans) from extreme susceptibility to skin cancer? A plausible answer is that postreplication repair which takes place immediately after irradiation involves constitutive enzymes which cannot readily bypass dimers but do not introduce errors. In contrast, at much later times, induced enzymes (see Radman, 1976; also D'Ambrosio, 1976) take over and synthesize straight past dimers in the template strand in an error-prone fashion. On the basis of this model one would expect excision proficient, but not deficient, cells to have removed a substantial fraction of dimers from their DNA before error-prone repair predominates. Furthermore, if Xeroderma pigmentosum variant cells were grossly deficient in an enzyme involved in the error-free closing of gaps, the efficient bypassing of damage may have to wait upon the appearance of the inducible error-prone enzyme system. The effect of caffeine on these variant cells would be explained if it further depressed the early closing of gaps by competing for the substrate of the early postreplication repair system.

(*iii*) *Miscellaneous Repair Phenomena*

Other repair processes which have been studied in human cells include the rejoining of the DNA breaks induced by ionising radiations and the photoreactivation of UV-damage. The medical significance of these processes, and any defects thereof, remain in doubt. In the case of ionising radiations, single-strand breaks induced by a supralethal dose of 10 krad can be rejoined at an initial rate of about 2000 per minute per cell (Regan and Setlow, 1974). None of the diseases so far studied show unequivocal evidence of defects in this rejoining process. In the case of double-strand breaks, it is not even known for certain if repair is possible in normal cells. Uncertainity also surrounds the demonstration of a photoreactivation system for monomerizing pyrimidine dimers in human cells. However, Sutherland, Rice and Wagner (1975) report an example in which strong photoreactivating light monomerizes the dimers induced by 100 $J \cdot m^{-2}$ of 254 nm light at the incredible initial rate of about 700.000 per minute per cell! Their enzyme analyses suggest that some normal cells may have even greater photoreactivating ability while some Xeroderma pigmentosum cells are totally deficient. Confirmation of these extremely important results is needed.

So far the discussion has been restricted to those DNA repair mechanisms which have been observed in intact cells, i.e. in situ. Another approach which has been used extensively, although with varying success, is to measure enzyme activities in cell extracts. As has already been mentioned, this has been done in the case of photoreactivating enzyme and deficiencies have been found in some Xeroderma pigmentosum cell lines and in one heterozygous parent (Sutherland and Oliver, 1975). Apurinic DNA endonuclease is another enzyme activity which is abnormal in some Xeroderma pigmentosum cells. Kuhnlein et al. (1976) estimate that the steady state concentration of apurinic sites in the DNA of cells in the A and D complementation group is some 10 to 30-fold normal because of this abnormality. Mortelmans et al. (1976) have shown the group A cell extracts are also deficient in the ability to excise dimers from UV-irradiated chromatin. These last results are particulary difficult to interpret because the data shows that there is a chromatin factor which interferes with the excision of dimers by extracts of normal as well as repair deficient cells. Extracts of human cell nuclei have been shown capable of excising γ-ray damaged thymine from DNA (Cerutti and Remsen, 1976) with the rates in some Fanconi's-anemia cell extracts being some 1.4 to 5-fold lower than in normal cells. A large number of attempts have also been made to purify the endonuclease(s) which presumably initiate the excision of UV damage in human cells but the results so far remain equivocal.

What clinical relevance can be gained from an understanding of the repair defects outlined above? Clearly, one has to be very careful in selecting criteria to class a DNA repair system as defective. The only unequivocal tests so far devised are those which demonstrate a gross deficiency in either excision repair or postreplication repair under in situ conditions. One can compare repair rates with the rates at which damage is induced by environmental agents and estimate whether or not sufficient damage is likely to remain unrepaired — or be misrepaired — and thus be a causal factor in the development of clinical symptoms. Ideally, one would also like to be able to calculate the probability of blocks in certain repair pathways channelling damage into a repair pathway of different error-proneness (Hastings et al.. 1976). The in vitro approach of assessing cell enzymes is of limited use unless one can ensure that the assayed activity is important in situ. Another problem in this approach is that subtle changes in an enzyme such as an altered K_m can have a very profound effect on the rate of removal of low levels of damage (KUHNLEIN et al., 1976). Even with more direct methods of measuring repair, however, the difficulties in estimating residual damage in the low dose range are severe and, until better estimates are possible, the exact relationship between repair capacities and the aetiology of diseases such as cancer will remain uncertain.

4. Clinical Aspects of Diseases Characterised by Defective DNA Repair

Three rare autosomal recessive diseases have been shown to have defective DNA repair as a definite molecular defect. These are Xeroderma pigmentosum (XP), FANCONI's-anemia-(FA) and ataxia telangiectasia (AT). Before summarising the main characteristics of each disease it is pertinent to comment on the problems of diagnosis. First, because of their rarity with somewhat fewer than one case per 100.000 births and considerably fewer patients than this under clinical observation, early and definitive diagnosis of these disorders is difficult unless the clinican is forewarned by the genetic history of the patient. Second, a definitive clinical diagnosis usually cannot be made within the first year or so of life because some of the important clinical features of these diseases only appear once the patient has been exposed to the environment. Another possibility that must be considered is that of other undiagnosed patients with essentially the same types of diseases but with symptoms (and DNA repair defects?) mild enough so that they simply merge into the general fabric of human illness. Indeed, one example of such a phenomenon has already been proposed by JUNG (1970) who believes that there is a disease "pigmented xerodermoid" of intermediate severity between extensive solar keratoses and mild XP, and in which the clinical symptoms do not develop until the third or fourth decade of life.

(*i*) *Xeroderma pigmentosum*

XP is the most widely studied of all the diseases characterised by defective DNA repair mechanisms. The major symptoms result from exposure to sunlight and first begin to appear within age 1 to 2 years, and include extreme freckling, telangiectasias and angiomata (even on unexposed skin), atrophic spots, superficial ulcers, kerato-acanthomas and warty keratoses. Within the first or second decade of life there is a progression towards basal and squamous cell carcinomas, and melanomas, all of which may be multiple in nature. Somewhat interestingly, it has been reported that these neoplasms are not always as aggressive as the histopathology might indicate. Nevertheless, death from metastatic epithelioma is quite likely in the second decade of life. (See ROBBINS et al. (1974) for general reference).

These symptoms are all the result of exposure to sunlight and can thus be controlled to some extent by the application of heavy sunscreens from early in life. XP patients may, however, have additional symptoms. Often small stature, poor physical development and low intelligence are cited and, in particular, the DE SANCTIS-CACCHIONE-syndrome which can include microcephaly, severe mental deficiency, dwarfism and hypogonadism. Cerebral and alivopontocerebullar atrophy due to neurone loss appears to be involved. (See ROBBINS et al., 1974)

Good evidence exists for XP having an autosomal recessive hereditary origin. There is, however, considerable genetic heterogeneity in the disease and those patients with classical XP can be biochemically classified into five groups, each of which is able to complement excision repair defects in the others (CLEAVER and BOOTSMA, 1975).
The exact biochemical defects in the complementation groups are not known and, indeed, as well as phenotypic observations of defects in excision repair, there is also enzymological evidence for varying degrees of deficiency in both photoreactivating enzyme (SUTHERLAND et al., 1975) and apurinic DNA endonuclease (KUHNLEIN et al., 1976). Positive correlations between these last two defects and clinical symptoms have been claimed. A further variant type of XP is found in a few patients who lack the early sensitivity to sunlight. In these patients the biochemical defect in DNA repair seems to lie at the postreplication repair stage (LEHMANN et al., 1975) although deficiencies in photoreactivating enzyme have also been reported (SUTHERLAND and OLIVER, 1975).
The one consistent thread that runs through all studies on XP patients is that all have at least one observable defect in DNA repair. However, the exact molecular basis of this extreme sensitivity to UV light is simply not known. Thus efforts to correlate repair capacity with clinical symptoms (SUTHERLAND and OLIVER, 1975; BOOTSMA, 1976) must be made with caution.
People who are heterozygous for XP seem to lack the clinical symptoms of the XP homozygotes — an observation in agreement with molecular studies which, likewise, fail to show any repair deficiencies at the cellular level. Only in heterokaryon studies which test the repair capacity of a heterozygote to the utmost, can some defects in repair be detected (CLEAVER and BOOTSMA, 1975). One in vitro study (SUTHERLAND and OLIVER, 1975) also indicates that photoreactivating enzyme levels may be lower than normal. These two observations suggest that careful in situ studies may detect subtle DNA repair defects in heterozygotes, and careful clinical investigations may demonstrate some sensitivity in these people. Finally, while discussing heterozygotes it is worth noting that the presumed (+/XP) genotype is not the only possibility; complementation may also permit (XP/XP') without obvious clinical symptoms.

(ii) *Fanconi's-anemia*

FA is a familiar aplastic anemia which is probably an autosomal recessive disease. It is characterised by hypoplastic pancytopenia plus hyperpigmentation, skeletal malformations, small stature from birth and hypogonadism. Microcephaly, mental retardation, deafness, strabismis and renal malformation have also been reported. There is considerable heterogeneity in the disease, and the age of onset of severe symptoms seems to be linked to some, as yet unknown, environmental factors (malnutrition, viral infections?). Within a given family this age of onset tends to be about the same and may be anytime in the first two decades of life. Most patients have chromosomal abnormalities which arise spontaneously and are largely of the chromatid type, e.g. endoreduplication, chromatid exchanges and gaps. Occasionally, these cytogenetic abnormalities may occur in the absence of other symptoms of FA. (For a general reference see LEWIS, 1974.)
The incidence of cancers, both leukemias and solid tumours, is very high in FA patients. No environmental factors have been directly implicated in these, or other, symptoms. However, one can argue in general terms, that many of the observed symptoms could

arise if somatic cells were susceptible to mutations or alterations which gave either a growth advantage or defect. Androgenic steroids have been implicated in the development of hepatic neoplasms in a number of FA patients undergoing therapy, but this sensitivity may also be common in other aplastic anemias (MULVIHILL, 1975).

Recent work has shown that as well as having a high spontaneous level of cytogenetic abnormalities, FA is also characterised by a high susceptibility to chromosome breakage by DNA-crosslinking agents (SASAKI and TONOMURA, 1973). This susceptibility may result from defects in the DNA repair mechanism(s) which act on interstrand DNA crosslinks (FUJIWARA and TATSUMI, 1975), while other molecular evidence indicates that defects occur in the excision of both γ-ray (CERUTTI and REMSEN, 1976) and UV (POON, PARKER and O'BRIEN, 1975) induced damage. The extent of genetic heterogeneity in FA is not known. Nor is there sufficient evidence to implicate deficient DNA repair in the aetiology of specific FA symptoms.

An extremely interesting facet of FA which deserves some mention is the report by SWIFT (1971) concerning the risk of cancer in heterozygotes. SWIFT analysed 102 deaths of relatives of 12 FA patients for which the probability of heterozygosity was greater than 0.1. He found that 27 had died from malignant neoplasm and that this number was significantly higher than the 17.4 deaths from cancer which one would expect in the normal population. Moreover, he was able to calculate that of the 102 relatives with possible heterozygosity, one would expect only 31.5 to actually be heterozygotes and that, of these, 15 probably died of cancer. Thus, the probability of death from cancer in a FA heterozygote is almost 0.5, that is, some three times higher than for the normal population. Needless to say, the assumptions and limited data render this estimate approximate, but even at the 95% confidence levels it does appear that in heterozygotes the cancer incidence rate is between 2 and 5 times normal. Somewhat independent evidence which supports this susceptibility is provided by the finding that the transformation rate by SV-40 virus of cells from hetero- and homo-zygotes for FA are, respectively, some five and ten times the normal transformation rates (TODARO, GREEN and SWIFT, 1966). This last phenomenon may not be connected with deficiencies in DNA repair which, in any case, have not been detected in the heterozygote FA carriers.

(*iii*) *Ataxia telangiectasia*

AT (LOUIS-BAR-syndrome) is the third autosomal recessive disease for which evidence of DNA repair defects have been reported. The two main clinical features are progressive cerebellar ataxia which is normally recognised about a year after birth and oculo-cutaneous telangiectasia which is seen by the third to sixth year. In post mortem it is usual to find cerebellar cortical atrophy but this does not usually involve the cerebrum or the brain stem. Apart from these two main features, a multitude of other symptoms are seen in AT patients including retardation of growth, premature aging of hair and skin, cafe-au-lait spots, and susceptibility to sino-broncho-pulmonary infections. Immunological defects also occur and in some 70% of patients serum-γ-globulin A is absent; moreover, there appear to be defects in thymus derived cells. Abnormalities in thymus and other lymphoid tissue are seen at post mortem. Some AT patients have a high incidence of chromosome breakages with rearrangements also occuring. A very important observation concerns the emergence of fast dividing clones of cytogenetically abnormal

lymphocytes which, in one patient, have been reported to increase from a few percent to 75% of the lymphocyte population in just $4^1/_2$ years. There is also evidence of cytogenic clones in fibroblasts cultured from AT patients. (See AMMANN and HONG (1973) and HARNDEN (1974) for general references.)
AT patients are highly susceptible to lymphorecticular malignancies and there is also evidence of an elevated level of other cancers (HARNDEN, 1974). The proliferative advantages enjoyed by some lymphocytes may mark a step towards some forms of malignancy but HARNDEN believes that the most logical explanation for the diverse disorders associated with AT would be in terms of one underlying basic lesion.
AT patients are known to be abnormally sensitive to ionising radiation. This radiosensitivity is reflected at both the cell (TAYLOR, 1975) and chromosomal (TAYLOR, 1976) levels. Recent evidence indicates that the basic molecular defect involves defective excision of γ-ray induced damage from the DNA of irradiated cells (PATERSON et al., 1976) — the exact nature of the deficiency varying from patient to patient with two complementation groups so far detected. As pointed out previously, the molecular analogy between AT and XP does not extend to the clinical level because of the very low levels of background ionising radiation in the environment.

iv) *General conclusions*

What common conclusions can be made about the effects of defective DNA repair? At the molecular level it has been demonstrated that these patients are defective in the repair of damage which is induced by environmental agents; at the cytogenic level abnormalities and sensitivities are obvious, and at the cellular level enhanced lethality is common (whether or not mutation rates are higher than in normal cells is still uncertain). At the clinical level, high incidences of cancer are evident — with the type of malignancy tending to be characteristic of the particular disease. In XP, the high incidence of solar-UV induced skin cancers tends to mask out susceptibilities, if any, to other types of cancer. It would be extremely useful to know if a completely sunscreened XP patient would have the same predisposition toward cancers as do FA and AT patients. In these last two diseases, it is possible that the clinical symptoms ultimately arise because DNA repair mechanisms do not act effectively on either the errors occurring DNA replication or the chronic levels of DNA damage which arise from environmental agents.
So far, only one possible outcome of deficient DNA repair has been discussed, that of neoplastic transformation. This is in fact probably a very special effect, possibly arising from a certain type of mutation (BOUCK and DI MAYORCA, 1976). It is well known that defective DNA repair can have a profound and detrimental effect on a number of cellular functions, e.g. alteration of metabolic events, loss of proliferative ability or even cell viability. Some such impairment of cellular function during development with subsequent amplification and eventual presentation as a clinical disorder may account for the neurological, blood, immune, skeletal, physical development, premature aging and secondary sexual abnormalities which have been recorded in one or more of these repair deficient diseases.
The crucial stage of development, during which DNA must be repaired efficiently, may be in embryogenesis. The symptoms seen in the repair deficient diseases, and the vari-

ations thereof, could well reflect two time related factors. The first is a build up of DNA damage at certain stages of embryogenesis either because repair capacity declines (Ben-Ishai and Peleg, 1975) or because certain differentiating tissues preferentially accumulate specific types of DNA damage (Margison and Kleihues, 1975). The second factor is the increasing probability of damaging a cell committed to a certain function in the future organism as the number of those cells increases. One would expect this probability to reach a maximum then decrease again once organogenesis and early histogenesis was completed (Wilson, 1973). It is particularly interesting that the effects of exposure to high doses of ionising radiations during early gestation include central nervous system and ocular defects, and also microcephaly (Wilson, 1973). Thus, embryos deficient in the repair of ionizing radiation type DNA damage (FA, AT?) could be especially vulnerable to such effects. Indeed, Petersen, Kelly and Good (1964) postulate that abnormal development of the mesoderm is a contributory factor to the clinically recognised symptoms of AT and Paterson et al. (1976) have suggested that this abnormal development may, in turn, result from defective DNA repair.

(*v*) *Do other diseases exhibit defective DNA Repair?*

So far only a small number of diseases have a demonstrable defect in DNA repair. Are more similar diseases likely to be discovered? Events over the last few years suggest that as we develop more sensitive tests for DNA repair capacity and as we understand the more subtle points of DNA repair, we will identify more diseases in which defects are present. Thus, in 1970 Cleaver examined nine diseases characterised by skin damage and, in some cases, sensitivity to sunlight. He found good evidence for defective repair replication only in the case of XP. More intensive investigations in the last seven years have demonstrated a repair defect in another of these diseases (AT), an abnormality in DNA replication which may also involve repair in a third (Bloom's-syndrome; Giannelli et al., 1977) and a possible DNA strand rejoining defect in a fourth (Progeria; Little, Epstein and Williams, 1975). This trend in detecting more subtle defects in DNA repair mechanisms is likely to continue.

5. Do "normal" DNA Repair Mechanisms Cope?

The assumption that the vast majority of the population have proficient and adequate DNA repair mechanisms deserves very close examination. Apart from the more subtle defects in DNA repair which are now being discovered in diseases of genetic origin, there is also some evidence for defects in acquired diseases. For example, a slight fragmentation of lymphocyte DNA in aplastic anemia patients (Hashimoto, Takaku and Kosaka, 1975) and some depression of DNA repair capacity in patients with actinic keratoses (Lambert, Ringborg and Swanbeck, 1976). Moreover, aging of cells appears to decrease some repair capacities (e.g. Mattern and Cerutti, 1975; Ben-Ishai and Peleg, 1975; Little et al., 1975) and, incidentally, also the fidelity of some polymerases (Linn, Kairis and Holliday, 1976). Whether these abnormalities in repair cause, or result from, other biological dysfunctions is not known.
Another facet of DNA repair in "normal" humans that has received little attention is the possibility of a *range* of repair capacities. A priori, one would expect any enzyme

activity to exhibit considerable in vivo variation from individual to individual. Proper testing of this prediction requires the use of primary tissue obtained directly from an individual. However, technical problems make tests with such tissue very difficult with the result that biopsy samples are usually taken and the fibroblasts that grow in culture from this sample are tested. Repair capacities of fibroblasts cultured from a wide variety of sources are surprisingly uniform with gross deficiencies only occuring in the rare genetic diseases mentioned in the last section. One cannot help but wonder if the highly selective and standardised culture conditions enforce this uniformity. Already, culture conditions have been reported to influence the levels of UV-endonucleases (DUKER and TEEBOR, 1975) and photoreactivating enzyme (SUTHERLAND, 1976) in human cells. Furthermore, the intriguing results of McCOMBE, LAVIN and KIDSON (1976) suggest that if the differentiated state of cells cannot be maintained in culture (and this is usually the case), the measured repair capacities are likely to be overestimates.

When the UV-stimulated uptake of tritiated thymidine by leukocytes is used as a crude measure of DNA repair capacity in primary tissue, a considerable variation is found in humans (e.g. a six-fold variation in 25 people; WILKINS and DAVEY, unpublished observations). Close examination of other workers data shows a similar variation (e.g. LAMBERT et al., 1976). Unfortunately, this particular test for DNA repair is open to a number of criticisms and the results need verification by a more reliable and quantitative technique. The problems in developing such a technique are outlined in the next section — suffice it to point out here that any mass screening technique for DNA repair capacity which was capable of measuring differences in individual repair capabilities and correlating these differences with proneness to cancers, or other diseases, would have enormous diagnostic, prognostic and aetiological value.

In this section the discussion has centred around "normal" DNA repair mechanisms. As a final comment, the point needs to be made that some of the severe diseases such as XP, FA and AT may have more widespread repercussions on the general population than their rarity would indicate. For example, in the study of FA heterozygotes, which has already been mentioned in Section 4 (ii), SWIFT (1971) calculated that 1 in 300 of the population of New York State were heterozygotes and that 5% of all acute leukemia deaths occured in this group. Thus, a slight preponderance of cancer deaths associated with a very rare disease is really indicative of a specific proneness to cancer in a larger fraction of the population. As yet, the existence of defective DNA repair mechanisms in FA or any other heterozygotes remains to be proven.

6. Prospect of Clinical Tests for DNA Repair

Any practical test for DNA repair capacity must be simple, repeatible and directly applicable to primary tissue (probably leukocytes). From the discussion in the earlier sections of this chapter, it also follows that the test must be sensitive enough to demonstrate small differences between samples. The best parameters to measure would appear to be the ability of cells to make endonucleolytic incisions (excision repair) and also to synthesise DNA (postreplication repair) after exposure to a test chemical or radiation. Measurement of these parameters reduces, in essence, to the problem of measuring the molecular weight of single-stranded cellular DNA.

Some of the tests with clinical possibilities are listed in Table 1. Many of these tests suffer from the disadvantages of cost, complexity or slowness. Moreover, most are only practical if they employ cells which are first cultured in radioactive medium to render their DNA radioactive. The simplest of all tests is to measure the stimulation in the

Table 1. Tests for DNA repair in human cells

Method	Cost (i)	Expertise (ii)	Time (days)	No. of tests	Prelabel Cells?	Comments
1. Alkaline sedimentation[a] (single-strand breaks)	++	++	~1	low	yes	sensitive but of limited use unless modified*
2. Chromatography[b,c,d] (altered DNA bases)	+	++(+)	$\lesssim 1$	low	yes	direct, moderate sensitivity, must know lesion
3. Equilibrium centrifug.[e] (repair replication)	++	++(+)	$\geqq 2$	low	yes	applicable to wide range of damage, lesions not detected
4. Photolysis of BU-DNA[f] (repair replication)	+++	+++	~1	low	yes	as for (3), yields somewhat better information
5. Autoradiography[g] (unscheduled DNA syn.)	(+)	+(+)	many	mod.	no	as for (3), somewhat qualitative, cytological value
6. dThd uptake[h] (repair replic. in leukocytes)	+	+	< 1	high	no	very easy screen, many artifacts may occur
7. Alkaline elution of DNA[i] (single-strand breaks)	+	+(+)	< 1	low	yes	not as quantitative as (1) but more sensitive*
8. Alk. plus HA chromatog.[j] (single-strand breaks)	+	+	~½	high	(yes)	as for (7) but much simpler*
9. Nucloid sedimentation[k] (breaks, untwisting)	+	+(+)	< 1	low	no	very sensitive, quantitation required
10. BND-cellulose treatment[l] (repair at growing pt.)	+	++	< 1	low	no	not fully quantitated

(i) Each + = piece of equipment costing approx. US $ 10,000
(ii) + = technician, ++ = graduate, +++ = expert
iii) low = less than 10, mod. = 10—20, high = greater than 20 tests per run

(*) Tests which measure single-strand breaks can be modified to measure either endonuclease-sensitive-sites or postreplication repair

Key for Table 1 References.

[a] REGAN and SETLOW (1974), [b] CARRIER and SETLOW (1971), [c] MATTERN et al. (1973), [d] IKENAGA et al. (1975), [e] SMITH and HANAWALT (1976), [f] REGAN, SETLOW and LEY (1971), [g] RAMSAY et al. (1974), [h] ROBBINS et al. (1974), [i] KOHN et al. (1974), [j] AHNSTROM and EDVARDSSON (1974), [k] COOK and BRAZELL (1976), [l] SCUDIERO et al. (1975).

uptake of thymidine in leukocytes and equate this with repair replication. Overall, though, severe criticisms can be made of this test on both the grounds of crudity and lack of quantitation.

Of all the tests available at the moment, the most promising is that of AHNSTROM and EDVARDSSON (1974). Cellular DNA is partially denatured in alkali then neutralised, sonicated and separated into double-and single-strand fragments on a small hydroxy-apatite columm. The fraction of single-stranded DNA in the column eluates gives a very sensitive measure of the original number of single-strand breaks in the cellular DNA. So sensitive in fact, that breaks produced by sub-krad doses of ionising radiation, the incision step of excision repair and the bypass of damage during postreplication repair can all be detected with ease. In a recent modification of this test (ERIXON, WILKINS and AHNSTROM, unpublished results) a simple fluorimetric assay for DNA obliviates the requirement for pre-labelled cells. The overall advantages of this method are certain to ensure its widespread use.

7. Conclusions

In discussing aspects of DNA repair which are clinically relevant, I have concentrated on the five criteria listed in the introduction. To this extent the discussion has been largely a scientific interpretation of the clinicans dictum, "observe" — "remember" — "compare". There are, however, many other aspects of DNA repair which deserve the attention of the clinican. Perhaps the most intriguing is the possibility of developing therapies to counter repair deficiencies. Of more immediate importance is the question of whether or not humans are exposed to agents which either stimulate or depress repair mechanisms. The role of repair mechanisms in determining a patients response to radiotherapy or chemotherapy is also largely unexplored.

Current research must, however, aim to establish the extent to which individual variations influence the efficiency of repair of environmentally induced DNA damage. This is the first priority in introducing the concept of DNA repair capacity into widespread clinical use.

Acknowledgments

The author is supported by the Cancer Society and the Medical Research Council of New Zealand.

References

[1] AHNSTROM, G., EDVARDSSON, K. A.: Int. J. Radiat. Biol. **26**, 493 (1974)

[2] AMMANN, A. J., HONG, R. (1973), in Immunologic Disorders in Infants and Children (E, R. Stiehm and V. A. Fulginiti, eds.), Saunders (Philadelphia) p. 236

[3] BEN-ISHAI, R., PELEG, L. (1975), in Molecular Mechanisms for Repair of DNA (P. C. Hanawalt and R. B. Setlow, eds.), Plenum (N.Y.) p. 607

[4] BOOTSMA, D. (1976), in Proceedings VII International Congress on Photobiology Rome, in press

[5] Borek, C. (1976), in Biology of Radiation Carcinogenesis (J. M. Yuhas, R. W. Tennant, J. D. Regan, eds.), Raven (N.Y.) p. 309
[6] Bouck, N., diMayorca, G.: Nature **264**, 722 (1976)
[7] Cairns, J.: Nature, **255**, 197 (1975)
[8] Carrier, W. L., Setlow, R. B. (1971), in Methods in Enzymology XXID (L. Grossman and K. Moldave, eds.), Academic Press (N.Y.) p. 230
[9] Cerutti, P. A., Remsen, J. F. (1976), in Biology of Radiation Carcinogenesis (J. M. Yuhas, R. W. Tennant, J. D. Regan, eds.), Raven (N.Y.) p. 93
[10] Chan, G. L., Little, J. B.: Nature **264**, 442 (1976)
[11] Cleaver, J. E.: J. Invest. Dermatol. **54**, 181 (1970)
[12] Cleaver, J. E., Bootsma, D.: Ann. Rev. Genetics **9**, 19 (1975)
[13] Cook, K. et al.: Nature **256**, 235 (1975)
[14] Cook, P. R. Brazell, I. A.: Nature **263**, 679 (1976)
[15] D'Ambrosio, S. M.: Fed. Proc. **35**, 1490 (1976)
[16] Dertinger, H., Jung, H. (1970): Molecular Radiation Biology, Springer-Verlag (Berlin)
[17] Drake, J. W., Baltz, R. H.: Ann. Rev. Biochem. **45**, 11 (1976)
[18] Duker, N. J., Teebor, G. W.: Nature **255**, 82 (1975)
[19] Emmett, E. A.: CRC Crit. Rev. Toxicol. **2**, 211 (1973)
[20] Fujiwara, Y. Tatsumi, M.: Biochem. Biophys. Res. Comm. **66**, 592 (1975)
[21] Giannelli, F. et al.: Nature **265**, 466 (1977)
[22] Harnden, D. G. (1974), in Chromosomes and Cancer (J. German, ed.) John Wiley (N.Y.) p. 619
[23] Hashimoto, Y., Takaku, F., Kasaka, K.: Blood **46**, 735 (1975)
[24] Hastings, P. J., Quah, S.-K., von Borstel, R. C.: Nature **264**, 719 (1976)
[25] Ikenaga, M. et al. (1975), in Molecular Mechanisms for Repair of DNA (P. C. Hanawalt & R. B. Setlow, eds.) Plenum (N.Y.) p. 763
[26] Jung, E. G.: Nature **228**, 361 (1970)
[27] Kellerer, A. M. (1976), in Biology of Radiation Carcinogenesis (J. M. Yuhas, R. W. Tennant, J. D. Regan, eds.), Raven (N.Y.) p. 1
[28] Kohn, K. W. et al.: Biochemistry **13**, 4134 (1974)
[29] Kuhnlein, U., Penhoet, E. E., Linn, S.: Proc. Natn. Acad. Sci. **73**, 1169 (1976)
[30] Lambert, B., Ringborg, U., Swanbeck, G. (1976), in Abstracts of VII International Congress on Photobiology, Rome, P160
[31] Lehmann, A. R.: Life Sciences **15**, 2005 (1974)
[32] Lehmann, A. R. et al: Proc. Natn. Acad. Sci. **72**, 219 (1975)
[33] Lehmann, A. R., Kirk-Bell, S., Arlett, C. F. (1976), in Proceedings of VII International Congress on Photobiology, Rome, in press
[34] Lewis, S. M. (1974), in Blood and its Disorders (R. M. Hardisty & D. J. Weatherall, eds.) Blackwell (Oxford) p. 1113
[35] Lindahl, T., Nyberg, B.: Biochemistry **11**, 3610 (1972)
[36] Linn, S., Kairis, M., Holliday, R.: Proc. Natn. Acad. Sci. **73**, 2818 (1976)
[37] Little, J. B., Epstein, J., Williams, J. R. (1975), in Molecular Mechanisms for Repair of DNA (P. C. Hanawalt & R. B. Setlow, eds.) Plenum (N.Y.) p. 793
[38] McCombe, P., Lavin, M., Kidson, C.: Int. J. Radiat. Biol. **29**, 523 (1976)
[39] Margison, G. P., Kleihues, P.: Biochem. J. **148**, 521 (1975)
[40] Mattern, M. R. et al.: Nature **245**, 230 (1973)
[41] Mattern, M. R., Cerutti, P. A.: Nature **254**, 450 (1975)
[42] Montesano, R., Bartsch, H.: Mutat. Res. **32**, 179 (1976)
[43] Mortelmans, K. et al.: Proc. Natn. Acad. Sci. **73**, 2757 (1976)
[44] Mulvihill, J. J. (1975), in Persons at high risk of Cancer (J. F. Fraumeni, ed.) Academic Press (N. Y.) p. 3

[45] Paterson, M. C., Lohman, P. H. M., Sluyter, M. L.: Mutat. Res. **19**, 245 (1973)
[46] Paterson, M. C. et al. (1976) in Proceedings of VII International Congress on Photobiology, Rome, in press.
[47] Peterson, R. D. A., Kelly, W. D., Good, R. A.: Lancet i, 1189 (1964)
[48] Poon, P. K., Parker, J. W., O'Brien, R. L. (1975), in Molecular Mechanisms for the Repair of DNA (P. C. Hanawalt and R. B. Setlow, eds.) Plenum (N.Y.) p. 821
[49] Radman, M. (1976) in Proceedings of VII International Congress on Photobiology, Rome, in press
[50] Ramsay, C. A. et al. (1974): Lancet ii, 1109 (1974)
[51] Regan, J. D., Setlow, R. B., Ley, R. D.: Proc. Natn. Acad. Sci. **68**, 708 (1971)
[52] Regan, J. D., Setlow, R. B.: Biochem. Biophys. Res. Comm. **59**, 858 (1974)
[53] Robbins, J. H. et al.: Annals Int. Med. **80**, 221 (1974)
[54] San, R. H. C., Stich, H. F.: Int. J. Cancer **16**, 284 (1975)
[55] Sasaki, M. S., Tonomura, A.: Cancer Res. **33**, 1829 (1973)
[56] Scudiero, D. et al.: Mutat. Res. **29**, 473 (1975)
[57] Setlow, R. B., Hart, R. W. (1975), in Radiation Research (O. F. Nygaard, H. I. Adler, W. K. Sinclair, eds.) Academic Press (N.Y.) p. 879
[58] Smith, C. A., Hanawalt, P. C.: Biochim. Biophys. Acta. **432**, 336 (1976)
[59] Sutherland, B. M., Rice, M., Wagner, E. K.: Proc. Natn. Acad. Sci. **72**, 103 (1975)
[60] Sutherland, B. M., Oliver, R.: Nature **257**, 132 (1975)
[61] Sutherland, B. M. (1976), in Proceedings of VII International Congress on Photobiology, Rome, in press
[62] Swift, M.: Nature **230**, 370 (1971)
[63] Taylor, A. M. R. et al.: Nature **258**, 427 (1975)
[64] Taylor, A. M. R. et al. (1976): Nature **260**, 441 (1976)
[65] Todaro, G. J., Green, H., Swift, M. R.: Science **153**, 1252 (1966)
[66] Wilkins, R. J.: Int. J. Radiat. Biol. **24**, 609 (1973)
[67] Wilkins, R. J.: Radiat. Res. **59**, 178 (1974)
[68] Wilson, J. G. (1973): Environment and Birth Defects, Academic (N.Y.)

List of Authors

BEER, J. Z., Dept. of Radiobiology and Health Protection, Institute of Nuclear Research, Warsaw

BENEŠ, L., Institute of Biophysics, Czechoslovak Academy of Sciences, Brno

DRAŠIL, V., Institute of Biophysics, Czechoslovak Academy of Sciences, Brno

GICHNER, T., Institute of Experimental Botany, Czechoslovak Academy of Sciences, Praha

GUNDY, S., Dept. of Dermatology, University Med. School, Debrecen

HAUSTEIN, U.-F., Clinic of Dermatology, University of Leipzig

HORKAY, I., Dept. of Dermatology, University Med. School, Debrecen

JACOB, H.-E., Central Institute for Microbiology, G.D.R., Academy of Sciences, Jena

JURAŠKOVA, V., Institute of Biophysics, Czechoslovak Academy of Sciences, Brno

KLUGE, K., Clinic of Dermatology, Friedrich-Schiller-University, Jena

KRÜGER, D. H., Institute of Virology, Humboldt-University, Berlin

MAGDON, E., Central Institute for Cancer Research, G.D.R. Academy of Sciences, Berlin

MEFFERT, H., Clinic of Dermatology, Charité, Berlin

MIKHELSON, V. M., Institute of Cytology, Academy of Sciences of USSR, Leningrad

NAGY, E., Dept. of Dermatology, University Med. School, Debrecen

POKORNY, V., Institute of Experimental Botany, Czechoslovak Academy of Sciences, Praha

PRESBER, W., Institute of Virology, Humboldt-University, Berlin

ROTREKLOVÁ, E., Institute of Biophysics, Czechoslovak Academy of Sciences, Brno

ŠATAVA, J., Institute of Experimental Botany, Czechoslovak Academy of Sciences, Praha

SCHROEDER, C., Institute of Virology, Humboldt-University, Berlin

SCHRÖDER, E., Central Institute for Cancer Research, G.D.R. Academy of Sciences, Berlin

STÖRL, K., Central Institute for Microbiology, G.D.R. Academy of Sciences, Jena

SVACHULOVA, J., Institute of Experimental Botany, Czechoslovak Academy of Sciences, Praha

TAMASI, P., Dept. of Dermatology, University Med. School, Debrecen

VARGA, L., Dept. of Dermatology, University Med. School, Debrecen

VELCOVSKY, V., Institute of Biophysics, Czechoslovak Academy of Sciences, Brno

VELEMINSKY, J., Institute of Experimental Botany, Czechoslovak Academy of Sciences, Praha

WALICKA, M., Dept. of Radiobiology and Health Protection, Institute of Nuclear Research, Warsaw

WILKINS, R. J., University of Otago, Dunedin, New Zealand

ZHESTYANIKOV, V. D., Institute of Cytology, Academy of Sciences of USSR, Leningrad

Subject Index

Bei Fragen zur Produktsicherheit wenden Sie sich bitte an:
If you have any questions regarding product safety,
please contact:

Walter de Gruyter GmbH
Genthiner Straße 13
10785 Berlin
productsafety@degruyterbrill.com